WHAT PEOPLE

Peace, Passion & Purpose has something for everyone—simply put, you will love this book! Kudos to Author Karla Mingo for her transparency in sharing with the world, the hurt and pain she endured, not knowing at the time that it would make her a strong and faithful woman of God.

—**Pastor Willie R. Johnson, MTS**
Journey of Faith Baptist Church
Red Oak, Texas

Congratulations to Mrs. Karla Mingo on her debut book. After reading it, I was not only amazed by her personal testimony of overcoming such insurmountable obstacles, but also personally blessed by the Blessing Lessons and thought-provoking questions she shares at the end of each chapter. I have no doubt that many others will be blessed by Mrs. Mingo's journey and "faith walk!"

—**Casey Thomas II**
Dallas Mayor Pro Tem

It was a privilege, pleasure and a blessing to serve as Editor for this literary masterpiece, known as *Peace, Passion & Purpose*. There's something very cathartic about shedding your layers and sharing your innermost secrets in order to be a blessing to someone in need. For this reason and so many more, I commend Author Karla Mingo for having the heart and courage to do so in such a unique and thought-provoking way. I have no doubt that her debut work will be a bestseller, as well as a blessing to the masses.

—**Angie Ransome-Jones**
Best-selling author of Path to Peace

An authentic peek into the window of Karla's amazing life journey of love, lost, and life lessons. This book is an invaluable asset to all who desire to become better not bitter and continue to live life on purpose.

—Shenikwa Bailey Cager
  National Conference Speaker
  Founder of That Wife Life

Darlene,

Always love God
love yourself and
love others!

Karla Mingo

PEACE
Passion
& PURPOSE

A Guide to Making Your Life Lessons
Your Blessings

Karla Mingo

Peace, Passion & Purpose: A Guide to Making Your Life Lessons Your Blessings
© Karla Mingo

ISBN 978-0-692-19969-5

Samone Publishing
P.O. Box 163
Cedar Hill, Texas 75106-0163

www.samonepublishing.com

Cover illustration: Creative Designs by TG
Red Velvet Ink

Editor: Angie Ransome-Jones

Bible verses reprinted from BibleGateway.com

DEDICATION

To my grandmother, Mineola Burleson, my Ma'Dea. You are now resting in Heaven with our Heavenly Father and there is not a day that goes by that I don't think of you and miss you. You were my very first example of what a woman of God should exemplify. Your loving kindness, servant spirit and unwavering faith are among the many things that I most admired about you and have tried to emulate during my life's journey. Everything I am today is because of you and it is through your life that I have found the courage to share my testimony. I love you Ma'Dea and hope that I have made you proud.

~Karla~

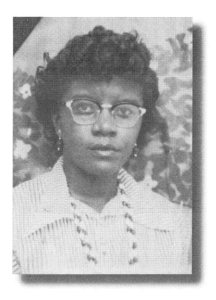

Mineola Burleson

"When a thorn pierces you, pull it out and use it as a weapon to win your battle."

~Karla Mingo~

WEIGHT ON YOUR SHOULDER

By Sydney Lewis (age 15)

The rock on your life
Holding you down
        down
          down

The feelings inside swallow you around
Pressure of the water during a drown
But you come to the surface
With a lifesaver thrown by the Lord

You still feel the wetness of the tears
As it runs down your face
Polluted with the broken pieces of your soul
Makes its way into the ocean we call Life

We've all been there
The feeling of being so torn down
Surrounded by so many people, but can't hear a sound
Your heart like a tree in the fall
Being so full of color and life until the leaves begin to fall

No mask can cover the pain of not being okay
We swallow the sad we feel
Feeding off the false reality that everything is okay

People look to something superior
As a way to not carry the burden of the rock on our backs
Bringing us down
        down
          down

TABLE OF CONTENTS

FOREWORD
BY KATINA BALDWIN

There is no bond like that of a sister, especially a sister who walks in God's light and speaks and acts in the ways of a guardian angel. My sister, Karla, is and has always been just that for me...

I'll never forget when our grandmother died unexpectedly, and I was overcome with grief and my big sister was there to comfort and care for me. She said in that sweet and calming voice she is known for, "It's okay Sis, you just need a change of scenery and a fresh start. Pack your things and come stay with me until you get on your feet." Years later, when I told her about some strange, unfamiliar physical symptoms I was having, she sat and listened quietly then said, "Sis, I think you might be pregnant so here's what we're going to do..." As I prepared to face the unknown, thoughts raced through my head about the anticipated judgment I would receive as an unwed mother. But when I caught a glimpse of my sweet sister smiling, counting on her fingers and calculating my due date in the meticulous way she is known for; it was in that moment that I knew everything was going to be okay. She was my rock during my first trimester when I became extremely ill, and she took care of me like only a big sister could.

It was my also my guardian angel sister who got me through the pain of rejection from my unborn child's father and reassured me with her comforting words, "It's ok Sis, I'll be right by your side." And she was. She got me through my delivery and even caught the first glimpse of my newborn daughter, Paige. Her words at the time still resonate with me. "It's okay Sis," she said, "she came out kicking and screaming and is feisty just like you!" Once again, I knew everything was going to be okay. Throughout my life, from childhood to my adult years as a single woman, married woman and a woman "unhinged" at times, my sister has always been there. She taught me long ago to give it all to God no matter what the situation and to always have faith and patience, and most importantly, to wait on His answer. I realize now that my sister has always been my guardian angel—always by my side, loving me, not judging me and gently guiding me and for that I am thankful.

I have watched in awe of her as she has continued to grow and persevere in any situation with the class and grace she is known for. For this reason and so many others, I am excited to see her share the wisdom God has given to her and that she has so often shared with me. I have no doubt that her book, *Peace, Passion, & Purpose: A Guide to Making Your Life Lessons Your Blessings,* will bless the lives of all who read it. Thank you, Karla, for being the best sister a girl could ask for and for helping me and loving me in every aspect of my life. I love you.

> *"You are my angel; you remind me of the goodness in this world and inspire me to be the greatest version of myself."*
> ~*Steve Maraboli*~

INTRODUCTION

Ever since I can remember, God has always spoken to me. Whether it was in my thoughts, my dreams, or amid my tears and prayers, His voice has always been ever-present in my life and now serves as my guiding force. Despite a lifetime of arguments, stand-offs and on-again off-again bouts with one another; our story is like one of those classic untold love stories and this book represents my long-awaited opportunity to tell that story. Early on, I knew God had plans for me that were bigger and better than I could've ever imagined, but my disobedience kept me from listening at first.

I'll never forget the day I was at my lowest point emotionally. I had just moved back home to reconcile with my first husband after being separated for five months. And while, in some ways, it felt as if a load had been lifted through our reconciliation, in many others, I still felt empty in side and knew something wasn't right. I was alone in my bedroom when it happened. Both of my girls were gone and I was sitting there flipping through channels trying to think about my day ahead. What am I going to eat this morning to tie me over until lunchtime? Should I take the 10:30 am class at the gym or wait to work out after work when he gets home? Then without warning, my heart started to race. I was overwhelmed suddenly and didn't know why. My breathing became heavy and the next thing I knew, hot tears were streaming down my face. Why God? I thought as I buried my wet face in my hands. I wanted to holler out, but I couldn't. I wanted to scream, but I was afraid. Surprising myself, I reached over; still sobbing, and opened my nightstand drawer where I kept my prayer journal, pulled it out and began to unleash my despair and frustration upon God, praying that he would respond.

September 18, 2003

Jesus, please help me! There's a big hole inside of me and I want to fill it. You are the only one that can fill the hole, remove the pain, hurt, disappointment. I feel hollow....

I stopped writing when I heard the soothing whisper that massaged my heart and caused my clenched fist to loosen.

"Your heart belongs to me," God said. "I can do all things. I will make you 110% complete. You will have a joy and a peace only I can give. I want to use you for my purpose. I want you to help me recapture the world. People are hurting. I need Healers."

Me? I thought.

"Yes, you!"

But I can't, it's too big.

"But I'm bigger."

I'm scared, I thought as I closed my eyes and allowed the tears I was holding back to stream down my face again.

"Fear not, I am on my way. People need to be saved."

Will you guide my every step and tell me what you want me to do?"

"Of course."

Will I have challenges?

"Yes, and you will make it through."

Feeling the sense of comfort that only the peace of God can bring, I set my pen down in the fold of my journal, closed it and clenched my eyes tighter; so tight that the tears had no place to travel.

What's first God?

"Let's heal you first," he said. "I have a master plan and if you trust me and let me guide you, you will have a beautiful life and your cup will overflow. You will be the light in someone's dark world. I know that you were mad at me for a minute, but I had to do what I did to get you here. You are so much further along than most people because you are now listening to me. I want you to teach other people to listen to me too. I am speaking to everybody, but they are not listening. They will never be fulfilled without me. I am the only way. You are right on time with my plans."

I thought I was being punished.

"No, that is not my way. I know your heart Karla. Remember, I created you. No matter what happens, embrace it with a spirit of thanksgiving and use it to become the strong warrior that I created you to be. As long as you keep me at the center, you will be fine...."

Chapter 1
MA'DEA

Train up a child in the way he should go, and when he is old he will not depart from it.
~Proverbs 22:6~

One of the fondest memories I have of my childhood was swinging on the brand-new swing set my grandparents bought me. Back then we didn't have the fancy wooden swing sets with colorful canopies like the kids enjoy now; just the metal ones with two swings, one slide and one monkey bar, and this one was all mine! I remember spending my days swinging on that old swing with my favorite red sweater-like cape that fastened to my head. This cape represented the long, flowing hair that I always wanted to have. Back then it seemed that I was obsessed with having long hair that I could swing back and forth and shake out of my eyes. The first thing I did every morning when I woke up was attach that red cape around my head. I would sit around the house with it, shaking my head in an exaggerated fashion every time I laughed. The funniest thing about it is that my grandmother, Ma'Dea, as we affectionately referred to her, didn't think a thing of it. Looking back on it now, I think she quite enjoyed it.

Living with my grandparents on their farm in Gause, TX from infancy until the age of ten, was one of the most memorable times of my life. My grandparents raised chickens, cows, horses, pigs and grew all kinds of fresh vegetables in their garden. My grandmother would feed us sliced tomatoes, picked fresh from the garden; garnished with her love and a little bit of salt and pepper to taste. Ma'Dea was a great cook, just like her mother; my great grandmother, Mama Jo. She made her own peach preserves, plum jelly, pickles and the best blackberry cobbler I've ever had.

The thing I most remember about my grandmother wasn't her salt and pepper roller-set hair or those strong, curvy hips that she carried me on some days when she was doing her business in the kitchen. Instead, it was her kind, gentle God-fearing demeanor and the way in which she served her church faithfully, that I most admired. Ma'Dea was raised in the Pentecostal faith, which meant that she kept her Bible close and went to church almost daily.

Being raised in the Pentecostal faith, I was taught to wear dresses and skirts, instead of pants and to don a clean, fresh face, as opposed to a made up one. Being as young as I was, these restrictions gave me pause. I remember asking myself at the time, *do I really want to be "saved?" I like pants and make-up and I like to dance!* It would be years later when I really understood that being saved had nothing to do with pants or make-up but had everything to do with accepting Jesus Christ as your Lord and Savior. My spiritual foundation was laid for me very early in life thanks to Ma'Dea. Every time she went to church, I went to church. I was always fascinated whenever I observed the ladies, and sometimes men too; dropping to their knees and watching their lips stammer as they belted out words and utterances that were sometimes unrecognizable. I was always there, watching and listening in fascination.

For most of my youth, I watched my grandmother serve God with humble obedience and servitude. My granddaddy, on the other hand, was the complete opposite. Although he didn't attend church on a regular like my grandmother, he was always very loving and kind, in his own special way, and extremely protective of me as his first grandchild. His name was Isaac Vernon Burleson, but everyone called him "Mr. Joe." My granddaddy had all kinds of tractors and trucks around the house like Fred Sanford from the TV show, Sanford & Son. In addition to collecting cars, he had lots of "side hustles" that brought in extra income for the family, like bailing hay. He also owned a makeshift gambling shack, a firework stand and a barbeque business. What I remember most about my granddaddy was that he worked from sun up to sun down seven days a week. I rarely saw him just sitting around. I admired that about him and believe his example led to my unrelenting worth ethic.

Growing up, I was questioned a lot about why I lived with my grandparents instead of my "real parents," but to me, my living situation felt normal so I was often un-phased by the line of questioning. My mother, Lura Burleson Hawkins was in her junior year at Prairie View A&M University, when she got pregnant with me, by my father, James Hawkins. They were both students at the university at the time so when my grandparents, being as traditional as they were, found out my mom was pregnant, they insisted they get married right away and so they did.

Not too long after, Ma'Dea persuaded my mom to go back and finish her education so that she'd "have something to fall back on." And so, she did and that's how Ma'Dea and granddaddy came to take care of me. Momma went on to earn a bachelor's degree in Education, while my dad went to work for an aluminum company. After serving at various duty stations overseas and abroad, he returned when I was around 2 years old. From there, he and my mother moved to Hearne, Texas, where they settled in and rented a duplex. By that time, I had grown so attached to my grandparents and my way of life that they knew it would be hard to take me away. Thankfully, my parents were comforted knowing that I was loved and well-taken care of; especially with the presence of my Aunt Erma and Uncle Bobby, my mom's younger siblings, who both lived there off and on while I was there.

When my little sister, Katina, was born two years later, once again, the natural progression was for me to move with my parents to be raised in the same household as my little sister, but I did not want to leave my Ma'Dea. Instead, my parents would bring Katina to my grandparents' house almost every weekend. The icing on the cake was when we got to spend our entire summers together. I've often been asked if I felt any jealousy towards my little sister, given the fact that she received most of my parents' attention throughout our childhood. In response I can say, without hesitation, the answer is no. Like hers, my cup overflowed with love, just from a different source.

I have so many fond memories of me and my baby sister growing up but the most memorable by far is the time I almost lost her; or so we thought, to an overdose of baby aspirin. Back in the day every parent kept a bottle of pink baby aspirin that tasted like candy and seemed to melt in your mouth. I remember one day my grandmother coming home to an open, empty bottle of baby aspirin and little Katina in a comatose state lying on the couch. My grandmother and Aunt Erma immediately sprang into action and jumped in the car and hauled butt to the emergency room. It was only ten minutes away but seemed like the longest ride of my life.

I can still remember my grandmother holding my limp, drowsy sister in her arms, rocking her, praying and pleading with her "no baby, please don't go to sleep!" As I sat in the back seat taking it all end, I became invisible amid the chaos, as I fought hard to hold back my tears. Inside I was petrified that my baby sister would die. When we arrived at the hospital, the doctors forced Katina's mouth open and attempted to force a tube down her throat to pump her stomach out. Their attempts were met by a suddenly lively child yelling out "Wait! Stop, I'm having a heart attack!!!" The laughs never stopped with Katina. Ironically enough, the woman I still call my "baby sister" is a practicing cardiac nurse practitioner and the story of the baby aspirin remains one of our favorites to this very day.

Blessing Lesson #1

I am a living testimony to the power of planting seeds in children early. The Bible says, "train a child in the ways of the Lord and he will not depart from it." (Proverbs 22:6). Growing up, everything that I saw and heard in church were seeds planted in my heart. My grandmother always knew that those seeds would someday come to bear fruit. It's the classic law of sowing and reaping—whatever you plant in the ground will eventually come up. I mean it when I say—keep taking your children to church, even if they fall asleep because the Word is being planted in their subconscious minds. As your children mature, it may often seem like they are not "getting it," but just know that they must maneuver the path that is pre-destined for them. They must experience their own trials and downfalls. As much as we want to, we cannot save our children from everything. Pain is a very strong lesson and is sometimes necessary, which is why God allows pain in our lives. He allows it because it will serve the ultimate purpose of serving His kingdom in some way. Whatever you are going through will become your testimony and will undoubtedly bless another—even if it's just one. If we had the power to fix our own problems, why would we need God? I have come to realize that the reason God may not fix our problems immediately is because He is up to something—He is trying to get our attention and take us higher spiritually. When God has a purpose and plan for your life, He will allow things to happen for His purpose, not ours, to be fulfilled. I had to learn this truth the hard way.

Again, my spiritual foundation was laid for me very early in life by my grandmother. As a young girl, I watched my grandmother serve God and be obedient. I was taught to fear and trust God and that heaven and hell were real. Sometimes we spend more time trying to convince people to accept Christ and to go to church instead of praying for them and being a true example of living like Christ. People are watching even though it appears that they aren't. Don't worry about your children who seem to have lost their minds or that husband who is still in the streets. Don't fight those battles with arguing, insults, complaints or moaning and groaning. Instead, we must learn to fight the battles we face, with a force stronger than any word a man could ever use—that force is the power of prayer. God's word is true but sometimes we have so much noise in our lives that we can't hear from Him. Think about it—we sit on six church committees and the choir, we have our three kids in two activities each, we're running four businesses, we're working out four days a week and work 40 plus hours a week. I'm not saying that there's anything wrong with any of those things but sometimes we fill our schedules so tight because being still is scary and uncomfortable for most of us. Being still means you must confront your fears, desires, temptations, your shortcomings, your pain and your insecurities. It is important to listen to the Holy spirit, but you can't hear it if you're always talking and moving. Sometimes you must be still and allow the presence of God to enter your heart. These things, I know....

THOUGHT PROVOKER #1:

What is the one thing or activity that you would be willing to give up to allow more time for communion with God?

_____

_____

_____

_____

_____

_____

_____

_____

_____

_____

_____

_____

_____

Chapter 2
PERFECTLY IMPERFECT

But the fruit of the Spirit is love, joy, peace, longsuffering,
kindness, goodness, faithfulness,
~Galatians 5:22~

When the time came for me to leave Ma'Dea's house, I had mixed emotions. On one hand, I was sad about leaving the only life I had known since birth. On the other hand, I felt a tinge of excitement and anticipation about the new life that awaited in "the city." I knew I would miss my grandparents tremendously but knowing that I would see them often gave me some semblance of comfort. My parents were settled and doing well in their careers now, so it was time for me, and them, to move on. In essence, my Dad didn't feel that I was getting a good education being in such a small, remote town and he felt that "city living" would be more beneficial and a natural progression into normalcy. But when it came down to it, saying goodbye to making mud pies in the driveway, sleeping with the windows open and swinging on my swing-set with my red cape blowing in the wind, was one of the hardest things I've ever had to do. What was even harder was saying goodbye to Ma'Dea and to my church home, Perry Memorial Church of God and Christ.

While I was sad about my departure and a little apprehensive about starting fresh, making new friends and adjusting to new surroundings, in my preadolescent mind, I also saw the move to escape the pain and embarrassment I felt because of some "incidents" that occurred, unbeknownst to my grandparents. I was around the age of seven or eight when I was

13

first touched inappropriately by a friend of the family, who happened to be female. Needless to say, I didn't tell a soul and pretty much blocked it out to the point to where it was non-existent. I've never spoken about it to anyone, until now—instead, I kept it buried deep down in the pit of my soul and in the very back corner of my psyche. Just the mere thought of it has always made me cringe, feel ashamed, guilty and nasty, even to this day.

As a little girl, I was afraid to say anything for fear that I would some-how be punished or blamed for what was happening. I remember on one occasion after an inappropriate touch, my pubic bone was sore. While I don't remember the details, I remember lying when asked about it after the pain caused me to reveal my injury. Instead of revealing my secret, I concocted a story that I had bumped my "private" on the corner of the coffee table. It was like an involuntary reflex and a natural reaction to protect my perpetrator, who was a family friend, and at the same time save myself from further humiliation and shame. When it happened a second time by another female, who lived in my parent's neighborhood, I became numb. As many times as I thought about revealing "my secret," even in my adulthood, I was never able to bring myself to do it and convinced myself to just let it go—*after all, what's the point*, I thought? Only through prayer and my longing to express my truth and finally tell my testimony, as God instructed me to, have I been able to speak on it publicly. Over 40 years later, it still brings tears to my eyes when I recount it, but I also know now that it is my duty to *tell my truth*—even if just one person is blessed by it and inspired to speak up and tell his or her truth too. With the growing number of men and women who have experienced and are still living with the scars of childhood sexual abuse, how could I not? I want people to know that whether in childhood or adulthood, any kind of unwanted sexual exploita-tion is not ok. In fact, it is a punishable crime. And while I've pondered in my head, a million and one times, what I could have done differently, I have forgiven myself for not speaking up. I know that this revelation will undoubtedly cause me to face questions that I may be ill-prepared to answer—like why I didn't tell anyone at the time or why I waited so long to tell what was happening to me? While I cannot explain the physiological effects that my abuse had and continues to have on me, what I do know is that *not telling* was a coping and protection mechanism for me and that it was just easier to bury it and pretend as if it never happened. My plea to everyone reading my words is to never judge a person that has been sexually abused. Why? Because the emotional and psychological effects are more complex than you think.

As I went on to live my new life with my parents and sister in the city of Bryan, Texas, the kids in our new neighborhood thought we were rich! We were one of the few black families that lived in a new brick house with a two-car garage; not to mention, the brand new, expensive furniture that adorned every room in our home. To add to the image, Momma drove a silver 1979 Lincoln Mark V that Daddy had bought for her. I can still remember sitting on the light gray leather seats adorned with wood accents and the smell of new leather dancing in my nostrils with every inhale. Daddy, on the other hand, drove a new burgundy Toyota Corolla, which made economic sense, since he had a much longer commute and wanted a gas-efficient vehicle.

When it came down to style and fashion, my mother was the epitome of class. She loved and longed for the finer things in life, and my Dad was more than happy to provide them for her and for us. Momma was, and has always been, a sophisticated and classy lady who loved beautiful clothes, high heels and all things glamorous. I remember her hair, nails and make-up always looking beautiful. Even with all the beauty and material things she was blessed with, she was always known for being humble and sweet and has remained the same to this very day. And while most people loved Momma, she had her share of haters too. Shortly after relocating to Bryan, my parents became known as a "power couple." Dad was at the club almost every weekend, but my Mom didn't seem to mind it much at the time. I remember how he would leave the house, cleaner than a whistle, with his knit suit, half-buttoned silk shirt, shoes that zipped on the side and a thick gold chain to compliment his physique. His afro was stellar in that it was blown out to perfection and his beard was always neatly trimmed. To top it off, he always smelled so good! Daddy worked hard and played even harder. But as much as he liked to drink and party, I never heard him use profanity, smoke or get drunk – even to this very day. He always made sure we were all taken care of and provided us with great memories including plenty of fun, weekend trips to places like Six Flags, AstroWorld and other fun family excursions. Like the typical father, he was also very protective and wanted the best for his girls. He had very high expectations for us and demanded that we conduct ourselves as the young ladies he raised us to be. We were expected to pursue higher education, become independent and to never rely on any man, other than him, to provide for us. He had a dominant presence in our home and as much as we loved him, we feared him too. But our fear was not a fear of harm or aggression towards us; instead it was a respectful fear that stemmed from our longing to make him proud and to never disappoint him.

I've always said that I was a good kid and my parents agree. I was always respectful and extra sensitive. In fact, I was that little girl that would cry inconsolably for just getting "a talking to." While my Daddy was big on being a provider for our family, he also believed in us being fiscally responsible and for us, that meant working and saving. I worked at McDonald's during the last 3 years of high school. Daddy required that I put half of my check in savings, he also allowed me to use the other half for whatever my heart so desire—for me it was a Dooney & Bourke bag, which I bought for $250 at the time. I remember being excited about having such a trendy bag and the mere fact that it complimented the passenger's seat of my new 1986 blue Nissan 200 SX, was icing on the cake. I was blessed with a new sports car my junior year of high school and my little sister, Katina sported a new Honda Prelude. But even with all the material possessions our family enjoyed and the perfect life we seemed to have, our lives were far from perfect because of a missing element—that missing element was religion. Even in my youth, I couldn't shake the unsettling feeling of not having a spiritual foundation in our home. At the time, I never questioned my parent's lack of church attendance or the lack of prayer in our house because I knew, based on some of their words and references and by the way that they loved us and others, that they believed and loved God and Jesus Christ.

When I was older, my mother revealed to me through casual conversation that although she was a believer, she and my father were "burned out" on church due to having to attend church all day on Sundays and several times per week. Still, I struggled with thoughts of my grandmother and how she so fervently served the Lord and even wondered if I would go to hell because of the way we lived. But as I grew into maturity and adulthood, the tug on my heart to grow closer to God grew stronger, which caused me to strengthen my connection with Him. Just as the Bible says, "train up a child in the way he should go and when he is old he will not depart from it," I can truly say that I will never forgot the teachings from my grandmother. In fact, all those years of going to church, Sunday school and Vacation Bible School, of listening to sermons that went on for hours and watching church members become filled with the holy ghost – all of it was ingrained in me. And despite my parents' lack of demonstrated spirituality in the years that followed my transition from my grandmother's home, I never once heard my Ma'Dea complain, judge or question them; instead she saw the struggle for what it was – a spiritual battle. For Ma'Dea, it didn't matter to her what anyone else was doing, whether it be her husband or her own children—she was determined to serve the Lord, to pray like a warrior and to love like Jesus Himself loved. She didn't hit us over the head with her Bible or shove the word down our throats but instead she showed us, by the way she lived her life, what a blessing and a privilege it was to serve the Lord.

Blessing Lesson #2

I was that child that never got into trouble and tried my best to do what I was told. I avoided conflict of any kind; so much so, that every decision I have ever made in my life was made with the goal of achieving peace—whether it involved a man, my career or even friends—any person, thing or situation that caused me stress had to go! I believed I could control my life's predestined path by the decisions I made. I hated disruption, problems, interruptions, and situations, like most of us do; therefore, I worked extra hard to avoid these things at all costs. In the midst of trying to create my own destiny, I finally realized that my trials were part of a greater plan that God had for me. I realized that my trials were necessary to catapult me to the next level of fulfilling His divine purpose for my life. I can truly say that my trials and tribulations have become my blessings. Because I grew up with an abundant of material things, I did not covet those things as an adult. Instead, my adulthood was more about seeking Jesus and the peace He provides; however, it can be quite the opposite for some—growing up without material things can cause a person to pursue fame and fortune over Christ. Nothing should come before God and I can truly say that if He doesn't do another thing for me, He's done enough. I've always said that I would rather live in a tent and be happy than in a mansion and be miserable. While I see and know many women who are enjoying the comfort of their big houses, driving fancy cars and toting Louis Vuitton bags, it saddens me to know that many of them may be struggling financially as well as in their marriages. Some are using alcohol and drugs to numb the pain, while others are having affairs and inappropriate relationships, while all the while portraying the perfect life on social media. My message to them would be to please stop pretending that everything is ok when it's not. Instead, try taking a real hard look at your lives and try to figure out what is truly important and what will last. Until you can stop and take a long, hard look at your life, you will continue to be like a hamster in a wheel going through motions, making little or no progress. Do you ever wonder why sometimes that you keep finding yourself in the same situation(s) over and over again? Why you start getting frustrated and angry at the world and wonder why you can never seem to catch a break? It's because you're trying to do things your way instead of doing things God's way. Try listening to a pastoral sermon or an inspirational CD instead of listening to gossip or negativity on TV. These are the things, I've found that help to inspire you and serve as a catalyst in creating spiritual growth and true intimacy with God. I truly believe that until you develop your own personal relationship with Jesus, you won't see the full manifestation of God in your life-you won't bear the fruit of the Spirit. Galatians 5:22 says "But the fruit of the Spirit is love, joy, peace, longsuffering, kindness, goodness, faithfulness." If I have all of that I have it all!

There's a whole new realm of living when you look at everything through spiritual eyes and when you come to realize and recognize that the love of God is everlasting. I put peace and God above everything. No longer am I defined by the car I drive, the house I live in or the purse I carry on my arm. I'm here to tell you that you can have all the money and "stuff" in the world and still not be happy. If you focus on Jesus first, He will give you your heart's desire. Pray over every decision you make. Allow God to reveal to you what He has for you. If you still feel wounded by any kind of abuse, God can heal you and make you feel whole and complete. The thought of my sexual abuse no longer brings tears to my eyes. I am emotionally healed not because I figured it out, but because Jesus delivered me from the pain! No man, no drug, no material thing will fill a void that can only be filled by Him. If you are holding on to anger at someone who hurt you, just focus on God and start building a strong relationship with Him. Talk to Him every day and tell Him what you need and what you want even though He already knows. Ask Him questions and then be silent. Pray with the expectation that he will answer you. It will not always be the answer you want, but it will be the right answer and you can feel good about it. When I was younger, I would pray and talk to God, but I wasn't as confident as I am now that he would answer me. I hoped that he would, but I had my doubts too. But the more you experience His faithfulness and obedience you will grow in wisdom. You will begin to pray, knowing without doubt that He will answer you. The wisdom I have now is not because I am 50, but because of my relationship with Christ and what He has shown me. You can be 60 and not be wise at all; they call that being an "old fool". You can also be 30 and have more wisdom that someone twice that age. And one thing I know is that you never fully "arrive" when it comes to wisdom. We, as the imperfect people he created us to be, will always continue to learn and grow as long as we are alive AND looking for our blessings through our lessons.

THOUGHT PROVOKER #2:

Have you ever been in a situation where you kept a secret to protect someone other than yourself? How did keeping the secret affect you? Did you or will you ever reveal it to anyone?

_____

_____

_____

_____

_____

_____

_____

_____

_____

_____

_____

_____

_____

Chapter 3:
ANGELS ENCAMPED

Be strong and of good courage, do not fear nor be afraid of them; for the Lord your God, He is the One who goes with you. He will not leave you nor forsake you.
~Deuteronomy 31:6~

I have always had a general mistrust of other women I acquired as a young girl, largely due to the mistreatment and "social bullying" I experienced at the hands of girls I went to school with—from elementary school through college and the sexual molestation. I will never forget the day in 6th grade that I was waiting for my bus after school when a girl named Rochelle walked up to me and hit me in the face. I don't remember much else about her except for the fact that she wore a jerry curl and that she hit me, for no reason, leaving me with a busted lip. This came out of nowhere and needless to say, I was devastated.

I was often called stuck-up, snooty, and bougie not because I was, but because I was extremely reserved and likely because our family owned a lot of material things. Some, not all, of my classmates assumed that I thought I was better than them, but in reality, I was just super shy. My experience being "young, black and blessed" undoubtedly shaped my mindset and caused me to be guarded and secretive about my life; particularly my blessings, for fear of the jealousy that would result. Therefore, every good thing or blessing that God bestowed upon me, I kept it to myself.

Even today, my circle of friends is small, and I tend to be selective with the women I choose to associate with. As crazy it sounds, I've come to learn the hard way that sometimes the people you think are your biggest cheerleaders are the very ones that are the most envious and jealous of you and your blessings.

In the Fall of 1987, when my parents dropped me off at North Texas State University (NTSU), which is now the University of North Texas (UNT), my guard was up but deep down inside, I was excited about the possibility of making new, lifelong friends and about being free! I was still relatively shy, so I didn't venture out too much at first, but instead, I always pretty much stayed in my room. It was easy for me since I wasn't allowed to take my car to school and because my roommate at the time was all about business. She didn't party or drink and always acted so responsibly and mature. As much as I wanted to spread my wings and live it up a little bit, she wasn't into that, which is why I was usually in our room chilling most Friday and Saturday nights. There was, however, one girl who I gravitated to her confidence and free spirit. For the purposes of this book and her anonymity, I'll call her Michelle.

Michelle and I really weren't what you would call close, but she liked to have fun; therefore, our friendship was inevitable. One night she wanted to go to a party on campus, so I jumped at the opportunity to hang out for a change. The party was packed, and I can remember feeling awkward as I maneuvered through the massive crowd of young, drunk teenage and twenty-something students. I was like a fish out of water, whereas Michelle was extremely comfortable, so I tried to assimilate as much as possible. When I finally tracked her down, she was talking to a man outside. As I approached them, I overheard him mention going to Dallas and Michelle agreeing with a promiscuous nod. When his friend approached, I realized very quickly that they were not students and were older than us -- mid-twenties, I guessed. In the back of my mind, I knew it wasn't a good idea, but for whatever reason, Michelle and I got into the car with the two strangers and headed South on I-35 to a destination unknown.

To this very day, I can't recall or comprehend my decision at the time; especially since I had always prided myself on being a "good girl," very responsible and the one who always made smart and safe choices. But in that moment, I threw caution to the wind and made a careless and dangerous choice that could have cost me my life. But God....

I still remember sitting in the back seat of the strangers' car and driving over Lake Lewisville. I didn't know if I would be raped, killed or worse so I tried to re-direct my mind and focus my brainpower on creating a plan of action instead. Michelle's intention was very obvious by the conversation with her "stranger of choice," so I prepared myself mentally for the possibilities. If the other stranger, or even worse—both, tried to force themselves on me, would I fight back? Would I play injured or dead? Would I let him or them have their way in order to save my life? I thought about Ma'Dea and started praying. I prayed for God's mercy and that I would make it out of the situation safe and unscathed. I had never prayed that sincerely or intensely before in my young life, but that night I bargained, pleaded and threw myself at God's mercy. Everything I had heard and learned in church engulfed my brain like a tidal wave. Scriptures started to massage my brain, old Negro hymns danced in my earlobes and the comforting spirit of the Holy Ghost ushered itself into my heart, providing an inexplicable peace.

Minutes after arriving and entering the mystery house, Michelle and Stranger #1 disappeared quickly into one of the bedrooms. Stranger #2 led me into another bedroom. I tried to throw him off by hiding my fear and apprehension; instead I acted like a willing participant—like I was "down for whatever." No sooner than we sat down on the bed, he started to touch me inappropriately. I quickly stopped him and asked, "do you have a condom?" In that instant, something told me it would better to comply with his wishes than to risk my young life. The look of confusion mixed with inadequacy on his face told me he was not smart enough to have a condom. In that moment, my bravery began to emerge. I boldly and firmly told him that I didn't engage in unprotected sex.

It had to be the Holy Spirit's intervention because without hesitation or anger, he simply said—"ok." Honestly, I think he was relieved. His demeanor and response told me that he was probably just along for the ride, just like I was.

We eventually got back into the car and they drove us back to Denton. Once I was finally safe back in my dorm room, I cried tears of joy that God had protected me from harm. This could have been so much worse. That's when I realized that the prayers of my grandmother had transcended time and I had angels encamped around me at all times. I knew without a doubt, that there was a spiritual component to my safe return. I used to question myself on why I did such a stupid thing, but now that I'm older and wiser, I understand that "All things work together for good to those who love God, to those who are called according to His purpose" (Romans 8:28) Maybe I was in that situation to protect Michelle from a gang rape or death, or maybe it was for me to solidify my faith in the power of prayer and to begin my journey back home to my spiritual foundation.

I would have to characterize the rest of my college tenure as uneventful in terms of the occurrence of any other strange situations. There were about six girls that I spent most of my time with, when I wasn't in class or studying. One of those girls was named Sabrina. Sabrina was from Dallas and would often go home on the weekends. She reminded me so much of myself that it was eerie at first. She had a quiet strength about her and although the other girls in our clique would gossip about her because she wasn't very social; I actually admired her because she was all about her business. As time passed we became closer and the other girls fell by the way side.

Today, I call her my best friend, and I am the proud Godmother of her oldest child. When she was diagnosed with breast cancer at the age of 31, I was right there by her side. I watched, waited and prayed as my best friend underwent chemo and lost all of her hair. As tired and weak as the treatments made her, she revealed herself as a strong woman of faith and fought the battle of her life like a true champion. Little did we know that she would one day provide that same lifeline or support for me as I faced the battle of my life...

The other college friend that had a lifelong impact on me was named Wytaine. The first day I walked into our Criminal Justice class, she immediately struck up a conversation with me and I instantly learned two things about her—that she was funny and sincere. Throughout the remainder of my college years, we became very close. We took the same classes and often stayed up all night studying for exams. We were adventurous in our own right in that we both enjoyed trying new restaurants on the weekends, shopping and just hanging out whenever we could. We always had each other's backs.

I'll never forget the time we had both stayed up all night studying at my apartment. We had an early morning class the next day, but when the time came to venture to class, I was too exhausted to drive, so she said she would come pick me up instead of me skipping it and jeopardizing my grade. By the time we arrived at class, I was sound asleep, so I stayed in the car and slept while Wytaine went to class and took notes for both of us. That was just the type of friend she was. When I landed my first job as a probation officer in Collin County a few months after graduation, she insisted we take a trip to Atlanta to celebrate. She was always there for some of my best moments, like being a bridesmaid in my first wedding. Little did I know she would also be the attorney to handle my divorce. In fact, we continued our friendship and supported one another for years before the good Lord saw fit to bring her home. I had no idea I would lose her at such an early age and not a day goes by that I don't think of her. When I do, instead of crying I try to smile instead and thank God for "loaning" her to me; even if for only a short time. Wytaine and Sabrina both taught me the true meaning of friendship; how to have a friend and *be* a friend, at a time in my life when I was vulnerable and guarded against letting other women into my safe space, because of the hurt and humiliation I had experienced in the past.

Blessing Lesson #3

The power of prayer was never so evident to me than when I put myself into a situation that could've very well cost me my life. As a young person, I had heard the testimonies about prayer and how it works, but it wasn't until I thought I was facing death, that it was truly real for me. For this reason, I truly believe that some lessons are only learned through pain and trials and sometimes you have to let your children bump their heads and wake themselves up. Some kids will learn the easy way, while others will learn through the experience of tragedy and trauma at an early age. As parents and loved ones, it is not our job to decide the life lessons they will have to experience in order to change their ways. Instead, we must equip them with the tools to be able to handle whatever they may face, pray for them and pray with them.

It's so important to expose our children to the word of God as often as we can, and to serve as living examples for them. I truly believe that the words of affirmation we speak over our children and young people will never come back void. And although we give our children physical life, we must also give them spiritual life. Every child is made wonderfully unique and although there might be that one child that just won't do right, he or she might have the biggest testimony and make the biggest impact on the lives of others. I truly believe that as long as we continue to plant seeds and water our gardens, that eventually our harvest will come about.

As a parent, I know it is not always easy to see your children make the same mistakes over and over, but the sooner you realize that there are some things you have to let God handle, the sooner you'll find your peace. Every problem we encounter in our lives is not for us to fix. Let me repeat that—every problem in our lives is not for us to fix. The more we believe in the power and goodness of God and embrace that ALL things work for good, the more we will experience God's overflow of blessings and grace. Whatever happens in our lives, we must learn to be thankful even when we don't understand why we are thanking Him. We must also learn to appreciate the people he places in our lives, whether they stay for a reason, a season or a lifetime. Even while in the midst of our trouble(s), we must thank Him and trust that He has a better plan. I know that it's easier said than done and I am a living witness because of my impatience. But I can truly say that God is working on me in that area.

In fact, I remember times when I used to get irate while sitting in traffic; but when I decided to start looking at things from a spiritual perspective, I found peace. Instead of getting mad, I started telling myself that I was delayed for a reason and instead I thanked God for the delay because I didn't know what dangers I was spared from by being delayed. He has always protected me from unforeseen dangers and encamped angels around me for my protection. This new renewed mindset has truly made my life so much easier to navigate. And when you start practicing this on even the smallest of problems, it becomes easier to apply your learnings to the bigger problems—and before you know it, nothing is a problem because you will turn every trial into your blessing.

THOUGHT PROVOKER #3:

Was there ever a time when a bad decision <u>almost</u> cost you something you love, or even possibly your life?

_____

_____

_____

_____

_____

_____

_____

_____

_____

_____

_____

_____

_____

_____

_____

Chapter 4
FAITH FILES

Trust in the Lord with all your heart and lean not on your own understanding; in all your ways submit to him and he will make your paths straight.
~Proverbs 3:5-6~

In the Fall of 1991, I found myself an unemployed graduate, with a Bachelor of Science degree in Criminal Justice. I chose this major because I thought it would be easy and less challenging than the other degree plans. My plan was to get a job as a probation officer making $2000 a month, which I considered to be good money at the time. It only took a few months before I was able to land a job as an adult probation officer and in my mind, my life was perfect. I had a good job, making good money, my own apartment in Dallas and a house full of new furniture—the only thing missing was that special someone to share it with.

At the age of 23, I met my first husband. For the purposes of this book, we will call him H.C. We met in a Dallas nightclub. I clearly recall my friend begging me to go out that night and as much as I didn't feel like it, I was glad I did. He was a kind and gentle man and ten years my senior, which I liked because it meant maturity and no drama. We dated for two months before he popped the question – seven months after that, we were married. As much as my friends and family questioned me about why I got married at such a young age, I stood firm on my decision. Although I loved and cared for him at the time; truth be told, I really wanted to avoid the hassles of dating and all the drama and problems that came with being a single woman in her twenties. I didn't want to go from relationship to relationship and indulge in the relationship games that people at that age so often get wrapped up in—I didn't have the energy or the patience for it. After being in the Dallas nightlife for a spell, that was enough for me to know that I didn't want to spend the next ten years of my life in that lifestyle, constantly searching and hoping. Instead, I was anxious to settle down and begin my life as an adult woman, a wife and hopefully a mother one day, which is what I had always dreamed of. We joined a large local church in Richardson. We were both very spiritual so joining a church as a couple was a given. Since I was married now, I felt that I could truly be "saved" the way my grandmother taught me. Fornication was now a thing of the past for me. I felt like that was the only sin I had committed and that now I could walk the straight path to heaven. Little did I know, no one really walks a straight path. So, one Sunday morning while attending church I was convicted to accept Jesus Christ as my Lord and Savior. I was 24 and believed that being saved would prevent me from experiencing the thorns of life, but like the old folks say, "just keep living...."

During the time we were dating, I remember being approached by a woman while I was having lunch with a friend. She asked me if I was interested in starting my own business and although I wasn't interested because of all of the other things I had going on, I knew H.C would be, given the fact that he had envisioned owning his own business. With that in mind, I took her card and passed the information on to my husband-to-be, which led to us attending an informational meeting and learned that it was actually a network marketing business. At the meeting, we met some of the sharpest, professional African American couples I had ever met; which impressed us both so much that we immediately joined. Without hesitation, we immersed ourselves into the network marketing culture and were encouraged to read positive inspirational books like "As a Man Thinketh" by James Allen, and "The Power of Positive Thinking" by Norman Vincent Peal. We were encouraged to listen to inspirational speeches by successful entrepreneurs while driving, instead of listening to the radio and watching TV. We built our lives around the concept of "garbage in, garbage out," and transformed our minds to speak life and positivity into everything we did. Instead of a honeymoon and family planning, we started chasing our dream of being financially free by building our network marketing business. Long weekends out of town and dumping paycheck after paycheck into our new business became commonplace. I begin to distance myself from my old friends because we were taught to associate ourselves with like-minded people only. My college friends were in their early twenties and doing what young people do at that age, while I was busy working and networking most of the time. Needless to say, our honeymoon never happened. In his mind, sacrificing this one "minor" trip meant that we would be able to afford to go on big trips to anywhere in the world we wanted to go! I believed it at the time, and although it never came to fruition, I have always been a hopeless romantic with the dream of flying off, with my husband, to all kinds of unknown, unfamiliar, exotic places with beautiful beaches and unforgettable sunsets. So, for the first six years of my marriage, I kept that dream on hold, while I focused on building our family fortune.

Although we spent thousands of dollars and most of our spare time with our business associates, we never achieved the level of success that we desired and never focused on "just us." My friends and family later revealed their suspicions of us being in a cult because of the fact that we were both so focused on the business and treated them like they were miniscule and secondary in a way. I didn't realize it at the time, but my family said I had changed. I had begun talking, walking and dressing like the ladies in the group who were older than me. I stopped listening to the R&B music I loved so much and started listening to jazz and inspirational tapes instead. In retrospect, I realize now that I played "the role" so well that I thought it was who I *really* was. I had become lost. Because I got married at such a young age, I never had the chance to be independent by setting goals and achieving those goals for myself and by myself. Whatever my husband said or did, I said and did with no questions asked and no complaints. All I ever wanted to be was a good, submissive wife because that's what I saw growing up—in my own household and in Ma'Dea's home, as well.

After four years of marriage we were both still working hard at building a business that was draining us of all of our resources and time. I quickly grew weary and frustrated because I was ready to start living the life I had planned with some semblance of fun and fulfillment. I wanted to quit the business, but did not want to crush my husband's dream and disappoint our circle of business associates; therefore, I continued the charade and one-sided smile. We decided to start a family even though we said we would wait until we were financially free, but I was sick of waiting and started to doubt that we would ever be as successful in this business as we had hoped. My first pregnancy ended in a miscarriage within the first month. I was devastated and depressed for weeks. I wondered why God allowed this until one day, I woke up and decided that this day would be my last day of feeling sorry for myself and that God knew exactly what he was doing, and I would start trusting Him to do it. Six months later I became pregnant with my first daughter, Somer. I was only 28 at the time but wanted desperately to stay home with her, but because I knew we couldn't afford it, I continued to work and pray about it at the same time. I also employed the skillset I had learned from the network marketing business by proclaiming my dream of being a stay-at-home mom and standing firm on the belief that the universe would make it happen. I had read so many books and listened to so many tapes about the power of positive thinking and believing in your dreams, that positivity and optimism seemed to ooze out of me.

Shortly after Somer was born in 1997, my husband at the time, got a new job and a hefty salary increase that not only supplemented, but was enough to replace my income. It was the blessing I had prayed for in that I did not have to return to work as a probation officer. Those days I spent staying at home, raising my daughter, were some of the happiest days of my life. For me, there was no greater feeling than being able to stay home and take care of my baby and not have to worry about having anyone else caring for her. I basically spent my days doing whatever my heart desired —from working out, to taking naps to play dates with other stay-at-home moms in my neighborhood. My baby was a welcome distraction in curtailing the lingering feelings I had of resentment for not being able to travel, hang out with my friends and have the normal life that I felt the network marketing business had deprived me of. Somer became my life, my joy and my purpose. Her birth also marked the beginning of what I call my "faith files." Because while in the back of my mind, I knew God would bless me, I was honestly shocked that he answered my prayer so timely, precisely and perfectly! This answered prayer became the very foundation of faith and testimony to witnessing the power of prayer and God's faithfulness. From that moment on, my relationship with God became more meaningful and more intimate. My mindset started to shift in a major way because now I believed that my life was good because of my obedience, faith and God's blessings. Six months after Somer was born, my Ma'Dea passed away in her sleep, but as devastating as it was, I was extremely thankful that she was able to see her first grandchild, my marriage and most importantly, my return to the church. She was truly the spiritual rock that blessed our family and kept us together, but now she was gone. I knew that someone had to continue that legacy and as much as the weight of that responsibility frightened me, I knew deep down in my spirit, that I had to keep her legacy alive. In her death, she had passed the baton on to me and I was grateful and honored.

After a couple of years of me being at home with Somer, we decided to build a new home across town in Desoto. We had lived in a two-bedroom townhome for seven years, so I had always dreamed of having a bigger space and my dream home. Career-wise, my husband at the time, was doing great, which allowed us to build that dream home I'd imagined off of one income. I know that it was my positive thoughts, visualization, prayer and faith and God that earned us the blessing of our new home. Like Somer, it created a welcome distraction from the resentment and frustration I felt from our decision to invest so much time and money into our business.

Unfortunately, a year after our move, things became a little tight, so I went back to work as an account manager for an insurance company. A year later, we decided it was time to expand our family, so in September 2001, I gave birth to our daughter Sydney. I was able to stay home with her for about 6 months which was a blessing because of the joy she brought, like Somer did, to my life. So here I was, 33 years old with two beautiful children, a 3,500-square foot house and a luxury Lexus, but I felt so empty inside. I didn't know why I was unhappy, but the loneliness and depression seemed to weigh so heavily that they created a hole in my heart.

Those feelings became so overwhelming that one day I remember the girls napping when I suddenly lost control over my body and fell to my knees in the middle of my family room. I started crying uncontrollably and crying out to God. I lay flat on my back, looking up at my 20-foot ceilings and double staircases, balling myself up into a tight fetal position wondering what was wrong with me.

"Lord, I should be happy, why am I not?!" I cried out.

With all of the material blessings God had blessed me with, I was still hurting inside and had a void that these things, my daughter, my house, or my car still couldn't fill. I began to realize that the joy and peace I was so desperately seeking didn't come from the material things, but I still didn't know what was missing. After all, my marriage wasn't bad; but we were more like business partners and demonstrated little affection towards one another. Six months after Sydney was born, I went back to work as a probation officer and had a flexible schedule that allowed me to work from home two days a week. This gave me free time to be able to work out and led to my love of fitness as a way of escaping the emptiness I felt. I worked out 4-5 days a week, was on a strict diet, became very toned and lean and at one point I even considered becoming a professional body-builder. I was extremely pleased with my accomplishments and as a result my confidence grew, and I started feeling like a new, sophisticated, beautiful grown woman. This was a turning point for me and the point where I started to feel my bravery and courage emerge. After ten years of giving my life to a marriage and business that didn't fulfill me, I told my husband that I wasn't interested in investing time and money into his dream of a thriving business. He said "ok," and continued to build the business alone; however, we continued to slowly drift apart.

After about two years of struggling financially, almost losing our house and filing bankruptcy, I decided that I would ask my husband of 11 years for a divorce. He was still sinking money into a business that was going nowhere. We had no savings, investments or retirement funds. We lived paycheck to paycheck. At one point, I even suggested we downsize our home, but he did not agree. We were no longer on the same page and I was fed up. H.C. was a calm person by nature, so although he was crushed by my decision, he didn't yell, plead or fuss. Instead, he said he would pray for God to change my heart. He never told me this, but I believe that he believed our separation would be temporary and that I would see how hard it was out there on my own, come to my senses and eventually return home. The girls and I moved into a one-bedroom apartment in Cedar Hill. Between work, pick-ups and quality time with them, I would frequent the local gym since I worked from home two days a week. After a few months of living in this small cramped apartment and struggling financially, depression begin to creep in. I felt like a bad mother because I had taken my kids from their dad and their home. I was confused and frustrated. I still wasn't happy and didn't have the money to get a divorce. My world became dark and lifeless. In the meantime, my husband was praying for me and the girls to return and willing to do whatever it took to get his family back; my heart just wasn't in it.

H.C. knew I was having a rough time and asked me again to come back home. In the midst of my depression and pain, I crawled back home with a deflated spirit and not a glimmer of hope. I felt unworthy, ashamed and embarrassed. I felt like my life was one huge ball of mess and it was all my fault. I started to experience feelings of grief that took me from a depressive state, to feelings of anger and bargaining. At one point, I even tried to bargain with God to give me clarity and understanding and to fix my marriage and restore me to wholeness. I volleyed back and forth from being desperate for Jesus to being angry at God. I was so deeply entangled in a web of anger, hurt, disappointment, regret, and unworthiness, and no matter how hard I tried, I could not pull myself up out of it. How did I get here? My depression became so severe that I was prescribed medication to help me cope. Although H.C was happy to have his family back together, I was in a downward spiral and the situation was even worse than before I left. We started weekly marriage counseling at our church, which gave me hope that God would fix our marriage and restore my peace. At the time, I felt that I was obedient; I did all of the things the counselor suggested, but the feelings for my husband that I hoped would develop, never came. One of the tools our counselor suggested to help me cope with my feelings was to start journaling. One day I was having a rough time emotionally, so I started journaling, which allowed me to release the anger I had towards God.

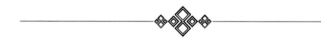

Blessing Lesson #4

There was a brief time when I was angry about how things turned out in my marriage and even bitter toward myself. When a door closes in your face, please believe me when I tell you to clap your hands and know that there is something better on the other side of your troubles, waiting on you. Just know that you are either being protected from something or being elevated to something higher than your wildest dreams and that the longer you stand in front of that closed door, the longer it will take to receive the blessings God has in store for you.

This chapter was extremely difficult to write because it brought back memories of pain, bad decisions and dark moments. But now that I have relived it, it brings me tremendous peace and I know that I am better for having gone through everything I endured. I have no regrets in my life and would not go back and change anything that I did or that I experienced. Pain is necessary to sustain life. Pain will make you eat, pain will make you change your ways, pain will make you get up, pain will make you sit down, pain will make you go to the doctor, pain will make you go to work, pain will make you go to church, and pain will bring you to your knees. But above all else, pain will make you seek Jesus. Pain is necessary for growth and purpose, and we should learn to be grateful for the pain we experience, knowing there is always a purpose behind it.... Always. The irony is that I chose to get married at a very young age, in order to avoid relationship drama. Never did I imagine in a million years that this decision would be the source of my marital woes.

THOUGHT PROVOKER #4:

*Have you ever been so frustrated or angry with God that it made you turn away
from him? If so, how did you find your way back?
If you haven't found your way back, what is your plan to restore
your relationship and intimacy with God?*

_____

_____

_____

_____

_____

_____

_____

_____

_____

_____

_____

_____

_____

_____

_____

Chapter 5
THE SAND BENEATH MY FEET

Concerning this thing I pleaded with the Lord three times that it might depart from me. And He said to me, 'My grace is sufficient for you, for My strength is made perfect in weakness. Therefore most gladly I will rather boast in my infirmities, that the power of Christ may rest upon me.'
~2 Corinthians 12:8-9~

September 15, 2003

God, I guess you have big plans in store for me. Well go ahead and work on me. I'll listen if you talk. I'll go where you want me to go, but don't expect me to be perfect. I can't do it. And how do I know you will come? And why did you allow all of this in the first place? What did I do to deserve this? Am I paying for the sins of my ancestors, will my girls pay for my sins? I want this to stop right now. The buck stops with me. Leave my girls alone, Oh, I forgot they are your girls too. We all belong to you, so you are in control of everything. But I guess I have no control of my children's fate. Well you know best. What will be their lesson be in all of this? Please go easy on them. They are so sweet. Don't let them hurt like me. Well, I do have to give you credit for bringing me home, that's one positive thing since I know home is where I belong. Now what? Let's go! If you want me to work for you then please heal me. Trust you? Ok. So, what do I do I the meantime? I'm still miserable.

"Stand."

How long?

"For as long as it takes."

Ok. But will you give me steps?

"Maybe."

I guess I'll hear you?

"Possibly."

What do you mean?

"Just stand and be still. Listen to your inner self and that will be me speaking to you."

Ok, I can do that. Now what?

"Just relax and breathe."

Ok. Where are you?

"I'm here. Always was and always will be."

Ok cool. So, when I ask, you will answer?

"Not always."

Can't you just pick me up?

"When necessary, I will."

I guess you'll take care of me.

I'll never forget the day I wrote this journal entry because I was at one of my lowest points in life and very angry at God. At the end of my conversation with Him, I put the journal in my keepsake box at the top of my closet, quickly forgot what God had told me and rolled up my sleeves to begin work on my marriage again, which I did for the next five years. H.C. and I did date night and became facilitators for the marriage ministry at church. I read books and prayed for my family and in no time, we transitioned back into what was comfortable for us, which resembled more of a friendship than a marriage. I tried, but just couldn't reignite the love and passion in our relationship no matter what I did. I honestly wanted my marriage to work and didn't want to uproot my children again, so I went through the motions and covered up my emotional wounds with band-aids that refused to stick. Despite my unhappiness with my marriage,

I continued to seek God and as a result, I drew nearer to Him. It was more important for me to be obedient to his Word than to abandon my marriage; besides, I knew I didn't have a biblical reason to get a divorce. I was terrified too that if I divorced this man, God would punish me in some way, not realizing, in my despair, that our God is not that kind of God. I had feelings of guilt about robbing my girls of a normal childhood with both parents in the home and also felt that it would be a selfish move that no one would understand or support me in.

So, there I was, I couldn't fix my loveless marriage, but I couldn't leave it either. I decided I had no choice but to stay. As a result, my inner light that shined so brightly before, started to dim and I became numb. I was 39-years-old at the time and had never been to a beach, which was a lifelong dream. Our finances continued to deteriorate and we had no choice but to file for bankruptcy. To make matters worse, I had not made the strides in my career that I had planned to make at this time. The depression started to set in again and I resumed my anti-depressants that I had put on hiatus while trying to rebuild my marriage. But that didn't help either. Instead, I grew more and more angry and frustrated with God because I felt as if I was doing everything He had asked me to, but he wasn't reciprocating with the blessings and healing I needed. I felt unloved and as if I had given myself to everyone but didn't get the return on my love investments and had never done anything for myself either. As a result, I tried on a bigger band-aid as a temporary fix—this time it was swing-out dancing. I had a female co-worker that I gravitated to at work. She would show me dance moves during breaks at work and I was so excited about my new hobby that she offered to come to my house and teach both me and H.C. how to swing out. I could tell my husband wasn't as thrilled about it as I was and was only going through the motions of the lessons because he knew it was important to me. Needless to say, the dance lessons slowly faded away and so did my hope in reconnecting with him. However, I was determined to do something that made *me* happy, so I decided to continue my lessons at a local club that offered lessons on Wednesday nights. H.C. seemed okay with it, but it just didn't feel right to me, as a married woman, to be out dancing with other men; men who weren't my husband. So eventually I stopped going.

As a result of giving up the one thing that seemed to make me happy, I slipped back into my depressive state. No one knew the depth of my sadness because I had learned to mask it very well like so many women do. We have mastered the art of pretending like everything is great when it's really not. And while this inherent ability as women to hide and push through our pain may seem admirable to most, I'm here to tell you that it is not what Jesus wants from us. He loves us too much. Instead, He wants us to seek Him and to learn how to replace the pain with joy that can only be achieved through intimacy and communion with Him. We were not made and put on this earth to suffer and there's nothing admirable about pain and suffering and being a victim.

My unwillingness to realize this led me to thoughts of suicide, because I felt like everything around me was falling apart and I saw no end in sight. I cried in spurts, without warning or reason and the first time the thought of suicide entered my mind as a possible solution to my woes, I knew I had to leave. I wasn't quite sure if it was the medication I was taking at the time, but the mere fact that the thought had even entered my brain, scared me to death and I was in a serious downhill spiral and knew I had to do something, so I decided that I would have to take my chances and face the wrath God for divorcing without a biblical reason. I was wracked with guilt over my decision because H.C. was a hard worker and all he ever wanted to do was provide for his family. So, who was I to destroy his dreams? But as much as I hated to and as hard as it was for me to do it, my survival mode kicked in and I was left with the decision to either divorce my husband or die inside.

So, after 15 years of marriage, and 5 years after my first departure, I decided to leave our marital home again, not knowing how I would survive or how much pain it would cause. I left because I needed to clear my head and figure things out. I purposely waited over a year before filing for divorce because I wanted to hear from God first. I wanted to be sure this was the right decision, so I intentionally kept other distracters out of my life in order to ensure I was thinking logically and spiritually. When you truly want to hear from God, you have to be quiet and still. Some women feel that they are not whole unless they have a man in their lives and afraid to ask God to remove that need. What I learned through my journey is that when you learn how to be in love with Jesus first, everything else falls into order. Believe it or not, being by myself felt just as good as being in a relationship to me because I felt free.

The first time I left H.C., I left with the notion that the situation was a temporary one, but this time around was different because I knew I would not likely be going back. With two daughters ages 11 and 6, I was in no rush to find love and had no interest in having a man in my life – no matter what the capacity. Others assumed that perhaps a "third party" had prompted me to leave my husband but that was the farthest thing from the truth. Number one, there was no man in my life and number two, this storm had been brewing for quite some time. In my mind, I honestly did everything I humanly could in order to save my marriage and salvage my family. Sometimes as women we jump out and in too fast, but I was determined not to take that plunge again. In fact, the first year of being officially separated, I deemed it as my time to heal, grow and rediscover me, Karla – someone I had lost along the way. I knew I had to be intentional about who I shared that precious space with and who I allowed to get into my head; whether it was my soon-to-be-ex-husband, my family or friends. I was determined that the only person I wanted to hear from was God and was hopeful that something miraculous would happen and I would realize, once again, that I had made a terrible mistake and return to my marriage. But that never happened. It was extremely hard to get past the feelings of guilt over my decision, which forever changed the lives of our girls. Imagine how they felt, waking up one morning to their beautifully decorated rooms with both parents, then coming home the same afternoon to a strange house and no father. I felt like a coward for not forewarning them and preparing them, in advance, for a separation that was eminent and for my own selfish reasons, I didn't want to face the pain or their reactions. Once we arrived at our rental home, I sat them down and explained the situation. Sydney, my six-year-old, seemed ok and wasn't too expressive; however, Somer was quite the opposite. She went into her new room, laid face-up on her bed and just stared at the wall for the rest of that evening. And while I did my very best to comfort my girls, the reality was that I had just broken their little hearts.

Needless to say, that first night I got little to no sleep and mostly cried and prayed to God to help me and my daughters. I prayed for peace, strength, grace and mercy and ultimately that His will be done. I also prayed for a clear conscience and for forgiveness for this "thing" that I had done. As He always does, God got me through the night and gave me the strength I needed to "put my big girl panties on" and to pull myself together and start walking in the prosperity and peace that He promised me. I started believing very quickly that everything was going to be just fine if I just stuck to my faith and clung to my Lord. I also had to change my mindset about God punishing me for this "thing" that I did. Instead I started speaking blessings into my life because I realized long ago that the words that come from your mouth are like seeds which can implant themselves into your mind, your heart and into the universe. The law of sowing and reaping is very real.

Only by God's grace did the girls quickly adjust to their new lifestyle and were able to see their father often, which provided more balance and normalcy. Thank God for their resilience and mine! Within a year of starting this new chapter in life called "Single Motherhood," I felt like I was finally starting to find my way and thrive again.

As a result, I started opening myself back up again to the possibilities of new adventures, friendships and opportunities. I was finally able to take the vacation that I had always dreamed of that I was either too busy or broke to take. I ended up forging a friendship with another single mother and together we decided to go on a cruise to the Bahamas. To finally see white sandy beaches and pure blue ocean was like a dream come true for me. It was hard to fathom that I was almost 40 and had never seen such splendor in my middle-age lifetime. Lying in the sun in my bikini, with white sand under my feet, sipping out of a coconut, was just what the doctor ordered for both of us. It was refreshing to finally have friendships outside of my marriage and business that allowed me to be who I truly was and had always been deep down inside. And although I attempted to reach out to some of my old college girlfriends who I had somewhat abandoned when I first got married, because so much time and distance had passed, I was never able to fully restore those relationships as much as I wanted to.

I was still working for Child Protective Services at the time, but realized very quickly after my divorce that the job no longer suited my needs. For starters, it didn't pay well enough to sustain my new lifestyle and secondly it was too demanding for a single mother. I knew I had to change careers, so I decided to get my teacher certification by attending classes four nights a week for six weeks. I specifically wanted to teach middle school because I wanted to help kids through, in my own personal experience, were the most awkward and difficult years to navigate as a kid. A few months after completing my alternative certification, God blessed me with a job as a 7th grade writing teacher. Within a few years after landing my dream job, I was able to build a home in a very nice neighborhood, which afforded my daughters a safe place to play and go to school. Another blessing!

After my divorce, I was not interested in getting married again because, in my mind, I was perfectly content with being single for the rest of my life. I had total peace of mind, a great new career, new home, new car and a drama-free life—so no thanks! And while I dated a few men after my divorce, none of them ever got very far with me because I was a very no-nonsense kind of woman and made it very clear that I didn't have time for foolishness. I had learned my lesson early on and became more dating savvy and "street smart," if you will, as a result. If a person did not add more joy, peace and love to my life, then they had no place in it. So, instead of focusing on finding a man, like many other women in my circumstances did, I focused on doing things which I loved, and which made me happy. Those void, empty and lonely feelings I struggled with for so long were finally gone. I felt whole and complete even though I wasn't in a relationship. That was such a beautiful space to be in and solidified my belief that only an intimate relationship with God, not a man, can fill the voids and wash away the residue of a failed relationship.

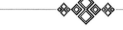

Blessing Lesson #5

In retrospect, if God had fixed my marriage when I asked Him to and waved his happy wand over me when I was sad, my testimony would not exist, my purpose would have not been realized and I would not be nearly as strong and grateful as I am today. I wasn't sure what it all meant at the time and why God did not answer my prayers to heal my marriage, but I decided that I would not let feelings of guilt and negativity consume me. I knew that God loved me and would make me whole again. I believed I would be happy and prosperous. I believed that He would protect me as long as I sought Him first. God has already written our stories and already knows the choices we are going to make before we make them. In fact, nothing surprises Him because he is the orchestrator of our lives.

Please know that I am in no way condoning or encouraging divorce as a cure for discontent and unhappiness. To the contrary, I am a witness that divorce is very painful and destroys the foundation of the family. Sadly, it's the innocent children involved who suffer the most. I hate divorce and whenever I hear that someone is getting a divorce, it truly breaks my heart. Believe me when I say that whatever you are going through in your marriage, if you just turn it over to God, He will lead the way. You must be obedient to His will and His way. While I know that everyone's situation is different, God is the common denominator in ALL situations, no matter what. We all have a pre-ordained path to follow, which God created—our only job is to walk that path *with* Him so that He can show us who He really is. But first you have to let it go and let Him take control. For years, I tried to fill my voids with everything from a new house and nice cars to having babies, working out and ultimately medication. In the end, none of those things filled the gaping hole in my heart. There's only one way to become whole and that's through Jesus Christ. It starts with having an intimate relationship with Him and then once you've established that relationship, becoming obedient to his Word. In my case, once I became truly connected to Him as my source, His will started to speak to me. For me, this message was in the form of a dialogue I started with Him through journaling. One thing I know for sure is that when He speaks to you, it will be clear, and you will know without a doubt that it is coming from Him.

Many times, we know God is telling us something, but we dismiss it because we're so distracted by what's going on in the carnal world around us that we become deaf and blind to what He is trying to reveal to us in the spiritual realm. There was always this feeling deep inside of me that I was supposed to be doing something HUGE for God. I knew I had a bigger purpose and that God wanted to use me in some way, but I dismissed it mostly because of fear of being stretched beyond my comfort level. When I dismissed it, it came back even stronger. You can try to dismiss it if you want to, but it's going to come back again and again. But there is no greater joy than when you are led to be obedient to His instruction and start walking in His divine will. Once you are in His will, nothing can stop you—He'll put the right people in your life, He'll open doors that you never thought would open, He'll clear the thorns and weeds from your path and He'll give you confidence and peace you need to sustain. I'm not saying that there won't be challenges along the way, but when you focus on the outcome and not the obstacle, your peace will prevail. I am a witness!

THOUGHT PROVOKER #5:

Has there ever been a time when you KNEW you were operating outside of the will of God? What did you do to regain your ground and find your way? Or what will you do if you feel that you are operating outside of His will?

_____

_____

_____

_____

_____

_____

_____

_____

_____

_____

_____

_____

_____

Chapter 6
SECOND CHANCES

Be anxious for nothing, but in everything by prayer and supplication,
with thanksgiving, let your requests be made known to God; and the
peace of God, which surpasses all understanding, will guard your
hearts and minds through
Christ Jesus.
~Philippians 4:6-7~

Four years into my singleness, I still felt at peace, content with my decision and finally settled into my new life. If I can be totally transparent, I have never been overly-ambitious; therefore, having achieved most of my personal and professional goals, I wasn't really interested in taking on any new challenges or changes. I just wanted to teach, relax in the summertime and have some semblance of a normal life again.

Although I had suppressed it for a while, I still had a passion for dancing so decided to resume my swing-out lessons since now was the perfect time to indulge. I started dancing several times a week and became very good, very fast. Dancing made me smile inside; it was intoxicating and gave me a sense of freedom that I can't quite explain.

Although there were plenty of opportunities to meet nice, attractive and professional single men, I decided early on that I would not fraternize within the swing-out community – I was only there to dance, plain and simple. The truth is, I loved dancing so much that I didn't want to taint my happy place by dating anyone in my new circle. Once school was out for the summer, I was able to dance several times a week and found myself with more free time than I ever had, since my ex and I shared custody of the girls.

With that, I decided to try my hand at dating again, so I signed up with an online dating service. I can honestly say that my intent was not to find another husband, but instead I just wanted a nice man that could add value to my life, as well as companionship. Instead of praying to God to "send me a husband," I prayed for His will to be done in my life; whether it be as a single woman or a married one. I honestly didn't want *anything* that wasn't from God Himself. I had total trust in Him and His will; after all, He had brought me through so many trying situations and had answered each and every one of my prayers thus far. I knew that if God wanted me to be married again, that He would send the perfect man for me. And He did.

I remember the day as if it were yesterday, I was sitting on my living room couch, scrolling through screen after screen of male profiles online. The girls were with their dad, so this was my way of entertaining myself in their absence. The moment I came across a profile picture of a handsome, dark-skinned man with deep, gorgeous dimples, I stopped dead in my tracks. I was instantly smitten so I took a deep breath and sent him an online message to see if his conversation was just as intriguing as his smile. After a few conversations, I realized quickly that I wanted to explore "this thing," to see where it would go. Needless to say, I was optimistically cautious, knowing that this man could either be the man of my dreams or my worst nightmare. But because I trusted God, I knew that He would quickly reveal to me whether or not this man was the one for me.

On the day that me and my new mystery man decided to meet, I decided to wear a pair of cute black shorts that showed off my legs, which were now nice and toned from all of the dancing I was doing. By this time, we had engaged in several great, laid-back phone conversations, so I decided the time was right to meet him face-to-face. I was apprehensive about having a formal "sit-down date" because I didn't want to be stuck out for hours if he didn't meet my expectations in person. I figured he felt the same way, so we both agreed to meet in "neutral territory," which, for us, was the Albertson's parking lot on a Sunday evening.

I arrived first, so I sat in my car trying to remain cool and calm, knowing the meeting could either be validation of what my gut feeling was telling me, or that it could be the moment of truth for both of us. By the time he pulled into the fairly empty lot, the summer sun was setting but there was still just enough light to get a good glimpse of him from my car. He drove a pewter-colored drop-top Corvette at the time so when he pulled up, I heard the sounds of Maze playing out of his speakers. *Now how did he know I liked Maze?* I thought as my heart started to pound a little faster with each breath.

With that, I took a deep cleansing breath and said to myself, *Ok, here we go.* I have to admit, I prejudged him based on my preconceived stereotype of men who drove fancy sport cars as being arrogant playboys who believed they could snatch any woman they wanted. I was never that girl that could be easily impressed with fancy cars and good looks. Instead, maturity and substance were my weakness, so I prayed, for his sake that he would come correct.

He stepped out of his car wearing jeans, a short-sleeved black button-up shirt and black loafers. In turn, I stepped out of mine, taking extra care to flex my leg muscles just right and swing my long black, wavy hair. Once he caught a glimpse of me and all my splendor, he leaned up against his car and crossed his arms. It was then that those deep, familiar dimples revealed themselves. At that point, I was fair game...

After our first face-to-face, Mark and I talked on the phone almost every day. But while our conversations were great, whenever I suggested us getting together again, he always had an excuse. At first, he blamed it on his work life and family obligations, but after a couple of weeks, he came clean by admitting that he was not ready to jump into a relationship just yet. He blamed it on his feelings of uncertainty and uneasiness about committing when he knew he wouldn't be able to give me the time I wanted and deserved. As disappointed as it was to hear, I said "ok," and kept it moving. Instead of being hurt, I was grateful that he had the moral fortitude to be honest with me. At this point in my life, I knew exactly what I wanted and was not about to waste my time with someone; with *anyone,* who couldn't give me the time that I needed, deserved and expected.

About a month went by before he started calling and texting me again. This went on for about two weeks with no response from me, because I had moved on and simply wasn't interested anymore. He finally got my attention with a text asking me to return his call because he had something important to tell me. I know it was nothing but God's divine intervention that broke me down in my stubbornness because before I knew it, he was on the other end of my phone asking me for another chance.

Among the many things he revealed that night, was a conversation he had with his father about me and how his Dad told him to follow his instincts and to come after me. I knew I was taking a risk by giving him a second chance, but I followed God's lead because I knew there was a reason for the reconnection, and because my God had never steered me wrong before. All of the lessons He had taught me at that point all ended up being blessings in the end, despite the pain.

Our first real date was as beautiful as it was romantic. He was a perfect gentleman, indulged me in great conversation and our chemistry was off the charts. It only took a few more dates to realize that our physical attraction towards each other was growing stronger; so much so that I felt compelled to tell him about my decision to remain celibate until marriage. I knew this could be a deal breaker, but if he was serious about me, nothing would run him off. I knew I would be perfectly fine if he decided to bolt, so I was pleasantly surprised when he responded with a nonchalant "ok."

I was at a point in my life that I wanted something real and authentic; a man that could be my best friend in life. For this reason, I was willing to put my requirements and standards out there without fear of losing. This strength and my attitude came from the fact that I allowed myself to heal and become whole again after my divorce. I became happy with my life and pursued my interests. I trusted God in whatever plan He had for me. That's why I was not afraid of being alone and of never getting married. Ultimately because I did not have that fear, I was able to stand my ground and keep my standards high. I worked hard to get to this peaceful state in my life and didn't allow anything in it that even closely resembled drama. I would rather be alone than to sacrifice my peace.

After "our talk," Mark and I pressed the forward button on our relationship and started seeing each other several times per week. It quickly progressed to the integration of our families into our courtship. I loved his family and he loved mine. He grew up in the church and was a prayer warrior, which I also loved about him, and his parents were very spiritual too. Growing up, I learned to make the distinction between people who truly "talk the talk versus walk the walk" when it came to religion and spirituality. But I could tell from his actions, that Mark was truly a man after God's own heart.

He was the type of man that would give his last dime or the shirt off of his back without being asked. He always wanted to help people and always made sure that the people around him were happy; especially me. He treated me like a queen, and I never wanted for anything as long as he was around. The more time we spent together the more we fell for each other. He loved my kids and I loved his, so eventually we started vacationing together and praying together as a family. I loved the way that he led me in prayer every night; even if it was over the phone.

There was not a doubt in my mind that I could have a life with this man, but this time I wanted to enter into it differently. Fearing that I would repeat mistakes of the past by alienating my friends, I made more of an effort this time around to nurture my friendships as much as I possibly could. At the time, I only had a few ladies in my life that I considered friends, but there was one in particular I was closest to, that I ended up losing in the process of building my relationship with Mark. As much as I tried at first to downplay our romance during conversations with her, it just didn't feel right.

For the first time in a long time, I was in a happy relationship and truly in love—so why should I have to mask that? Why couldn't she be happy for me? I would've been happy for her. It took an awkward and abrupt end to our friendship to make me realize that everyone in our lives is not meant to be there forever. There is definitely something to the old cliché that people will exist in our lives for either a reason, a season or a lifetime and once we truly begin to grasp that concept, it becomes easier for us to accept when those relationships and friendships end. Once you train your mind and heart to believe in the blessings behind the lessons, life becomes sweeter than we could ever imagine.

A couple of years into the relationship, Mark finally popped the question. But it wasn't quite the question I wanted him to ask. He asked me if I wanted a promise ring. I looked at him in bewilderment and politely responded, "no thank you."

We can laugh about it now, but my thought process at the time (even now) is that promise rings are for girls and engagement rings are for women. I wasn't that girl that ever wanted to nag or give marriage ultimatums, because I was happy with the way things were and had faith that when the time was right, we would both know it.

After four years of happily dating, we realized that we were both fast-approaching our fifties and both of us seemed to be growing weary of asking that all-to-familiar question—*your house or mine?* One Friday evening in February 2016, Mark asked me to meet him at a jewelry store. My first thought was, *is this brotha' looking at promise rings again or is this a Valentine's Day gift?*

When I arrived, he smiled, kissed me on my forehead and asked me to pick out the engagement ring of my choice. He never officially asked me to marry him, but I was just as thrilled as if I was standing at the base of the Eiffel Tower with the man of my dreams, which was Mark, on bended knee. It was the perfect ending to a chapter we both agreed was time to close. I was excited to start a new chapter in my life.

Although I was excited about the wedding date, which we set for May 17, 2017, I was even more thrilled about the honeymoon. Going to Hawaii was at the top of my bucket list and I was finally getting the chance to travel to paradise with my best friend, who also happened to be the love of my life.

I spent weeks looking for the perfect venue and hours online looking for flights along with hotels in Hawaii because our honeymoon *had* to be perfect. The plan was to get married that Saturday and head to our beautiful honeymoon destination that Sunday.

My dream was finally coming true. In fact, I remember feeling at the time like my life was like a continuous dream, and I was completely and blissfully thankful for it. I had no problems—no relationship problems, no money problems, no career problems, no health problems and no family problems. Thanking God for every blessing was a habitual practice for me because I knew that every good thing in my life, including Mark, came from Him.

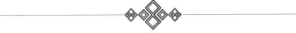

Blessing Lesson #6

Although I do not profess to be a relationship expert, here is what I do know:

1. **You are a Queen.**

    For our first date, Mark chose a seafood restaurant in his area that was in the opposite direction of where I lived. He suggested we should meet there. I told him without hesitation, that I wanted him to come pick me up because I should not have to drive. I could hear the hesitation in his voice, but he agreed. Another climb up the pedestal. For me, I needed to know if he was serious about me. I didn't care how far he had to drive, because a man will drive as far as he has to if he really wants you. Ladies, stop making things so easy for men. Some ladies are driving across town to see a man and he has never come to you. You in your car more than him. Chivalry is not dead, women have taken the option away from men by doing it all themselves and they will let you do it. Let them work for it. Believe it or not they prefer to work for it because it has more value.

2. **Grow closer and pray to Him for His will for your life, not yours.**

Seek Him with all of your heart. Ask God what His purpose is for you. Ask him to illuminate the path he has for you. Work on your relationship with Jesus, so that when you are approached by a man, you will be able to feel his spirit first and recognize what's good and what isn't. Girlfriends can be very powerful because they were there before that man and we think they always have our best interest at heart. There are many ladies that have lost good men, listening to a girlfriend and taking her advice. It's ok to seek advice but be able to discern for yourself. Sometimes the person closest to you is secretly hoping you would fail. Ladies, there will come a time when you need to stop talking to your girlfriends about your relationships. Talk to women who have fruit. Talk to God-fearing women who have successful marriages. Be very selective on who you allow in your inner circle and into your business.

3. **Speak positively over everything in your life.**

Basically, I believed with all of my heart that regardless of how many people tell me about the low-down, no-good men out there, I knew there were some great men and that there was one man in this world that was perfect for me. I knew God could bless me with my heart's desire regardless of what's seen in the natural. I knew God had supernatural powers and if He wanted me to be married, and I trusted Him, he would send the perfect person to me. Sometimes we are where we are because of the friends we listen to. If you are associating yourself with friends who are always talking about what they don't have or what they can't get, or how hard it is, then you need some new friends. If you're not careful, you will end up thinking and speaking like your negative peers and wonder why you are not seeing your blessings. What you think and what you speak are very powerful tools to creating the life that you want. I believe you block your blessing with the words that you speak. It doesn't matter what it looks like through the human eye, you have to look at life through spiritual eyes.

4. **Fall in love with yourself.**

   When you act like a queen, you will be treated as such. Don't lower your standards to get a man. A man can tell immediately what kind of woman you are by your expectations at the beginning. I get the fact that women are strong, independent and making their own coins. We own businesses and have achieved a lot of success. Yes, you can do it all by yourself, but let a man be what God created him to be, a leader. Trust me, we have more power than you know. You will never lose your power by letting a man take care of you. Let him drive, let him pay, let him open the door, let him pull out the chair. Expect that from day 1. If he's the one for you, he isn't going anywhere, if he runs, clap your hands. This will allow you to keep space open for the man that God has for you. If you keep dealing with "men not ready," there's no room for "the one who's ready" to come in. Some ladies are hanging on to a piece of a man while the whole man God has for you is waiting for his opening. Don't be desperate for any human. Humans are flawed and will let you down. They will disappoint you. Be desperate for Jesus and you will have continuous joy regardless of the human disappointments in your life.

5. To love is to sacrifice.

Mark never said anything to me about it or ever asked me to stop dancing. Without saying anything to him, I decided to step away from dancing (no pun intended). I understood how this would eventually affect our relationship and decided on what's more important right now and where I wanted to go. I could have stood my ground and kept dancing, but sometimes you have to sacrifice for something greater. That didn't make me weak as a woman. It made us stronger as a couple. He also stopped going to the club without me asking him. Ladies stop doing things to create dissention in your relationships. If you want a strong relationship and marriage, you have to give up some things you did as a single woman, and he shouldn't have to ask you. You can still be independent and do your thing, just make sure you are both on the same page and both feel good about it. If you want him to climb that pedestal and get you, you have to give him something to climb for. I made the right decision and have no regrets.

6. God wants the best for you.

One thing I know for sure, when a man is interested in you, he will find time to be with you. We can be so desperate for a man that we will tolerate and believe almost anything they tell us. Ladies, put yourself on a high pedestal and make a man climb it to get to you. Women are beautiful queens and should be treated as such. Love yourself so much that you never allow yourself to be mistreated by a man. The way a man treats you is based on your expectations. He will only do to you what you allow him to do. You are a prize to be won, and he needs to know that from day one. I'm not saying to be arrogant or act like you're too good for someone, but be confident in who you are and what you bring to the table. You will save yourself a lot of heartache if you remember that God wants the best for you, and if what's standing in front of you is not aligning with that purpose, then keep moving. Don't let a man string you along with empty promises. For those of you who never had a father or male role model to show you love and how to be treated, it's ok because you have a heavenly father that has loved and treated you better than any human being.

THOUGHT PROVOKER #6:

Have you ever felt so much at peace that it scared you? What does peace look and feel like for you? Is it sleeping through the night, is it being free from worry, is it having the perfect relationship or dream job? Where do you find peace? And if you don't have peace, how will you start trying to achieve it today?

_____

_____

_____

_____

_____

_____

_____

_____

_____

_____

_____

_____

_____

_____

Chapter 7
INTO THE WILDERNESS

No weapon formed against you shall prosper, And every tongue which rises against you in judgment You shall condemn. This is the heritage of the servants of the Lord And their righteousness is from Me, Says the Lord."
~Isaiah 54:17~

As if planning my dream wedding to the man of my dreams wasn't a blessing in itself, I was doing great in my career and had just received a promotion at work. Mark was doing remarkably well too. His 27 years of experience in the car business was beginning to pay off in a major way —another dealership offered him a tremendous opportunity in management with a salary increase to match. We both felt as if we were "living the dream," and genuinely grateful for it.

It was a night in January 2017, as I laid in bed relaxing and watching TV that my life was forever changed. My bra was usually the first thing that came off when I got home every night after a long day at work. Being the full-breasted 34DD that I was and had been since high school, I had always looked forward to the exhilaration of letting "my girls" loose every night. So, as I lay there relaxed, I caressed the impression in my skin where my bra was positioned earlier in the day. As my fingertips scaled the area just below my nipple on my left breast, I noticed an area that felt different; a nodule I had never noticed before. I immediately sat up in my bed and pressed harder around the area surrounding my left nipple, calmly trying to locate "it." Much to my shock, "it" turned out to be a lump that was implanted inconspicuously just above my left nipple. It was very small and subtle but felt like the size of a marble. I didn't panic at first since the lump was so small and wasn't prominent or protruding.

At this point, I still wasn't sure if it was just part of the normal lumpiness of my breast or something I should really be concerned about, so I went to bed praying that it wouldn't be there in the morning. The next morning "it" was still there; in the same spot, feeling the same way it felt the night before. As you can imagine, a barrage of thoughts started to flood my brain —thoughts of chemo, radiation, mastectomies, sickness, hair loss—you name it, I thought it. There were so many "what ifs" in my head that I knew I had to control them quickly and replace them with positive, optimistic, faithful thoughts—so I began to draw from my "Faith Files" like I had always done in the past. I found peace in recalling all of the trials and tribulations that God had brought me through in the past, which were too many to count. I went into an inherent posture of prayer and started speaking life into my body and into my mind. I told myself that whatever "it" was, that it would be alright. I didn't tell any of my family members about the lump because I didn't want them to worry; however, I did casually mention to Mark that I had found a lump in my breast but that it was probably nothing. He was calm about it, reassured me that it would be okay but urged me to get it checked out as soon as possible. He even offered to go with me.

Prior to this incident, I had always been pretty good about staying on track with my annual well-woman exams and mammograms. And as many times as I thought about skipping them in the past, I always imagined that the one I skipped would be the one something would be wrong; therefore, I never wanted to take that risk so I never missed one. Due to some insurance changes at my job, there was a coverage change that took effect in the new school year, which meant that the clinic I had previously frequented was no longer a qualifying provider under my new plan. I had every intention of finding a new provider and scheduling my annual exam but had not gotten around to it, due to my promotion and heavier workload. In full transparency, I just never made it a priority. While I knew that monthly breast exams were recommended, I only self-examined once, maybe twice a year and only when I was reminded or prompted to do so when another friend or friend of a friend was diagnosed. My call to the new provider to schedule my mammogram resulted in a referral to my OB/GYN who, in turn, had to give me another referral for a mammogram. Unfortunately, because my insurance had changed, I had to find a new OB/GYN as well. It took me only a couple of hours and a few phone calls to find one, only to find that the first availability for a new patient appointment was not until February, which was 1 month away. My heart sank. *This can't be happening right now,* I thought to myself. Our wedding was four months away. The venue and the honeymoon had been booked. I was in the process of looking at caterers and dresses. Mark and I were so happy and had been so blessed—life was too good for this to be happening. Once again, I started training my brain to think positive thoughts. As I patiently waited for my appointment date, I searched the internet for anything and everything I could find on breast cancer. I was somewhat relieved to find that there were several known reasons, other than cancer, for breast lumps. My faith told me that mine was in the "other" category so with that I began journaling my experience in what I now call "My Breast Notes."

On the day of my ultrasound, I was prepared, prayed up and felt like I was a semi-expert on all things related to breast cancer. I had done extensive online research on what a malignant and non-malignant tumor looked like; even to the point where I felt like I could recognize it on my own ultrasound. While lying on the table during my procedure, I asked if I could look at the screen. To my terror, I instantly saw the tumor on the screen and recognized the characteristics of a malignant tumor. Of course, the nurse couldn't disclose any information or even give me her opinion, but her energy told me that she recognized it too. Sensing my energy, she grabbed my hand and said, "Listen, honey, you are going to be just fine regardless of the results. Look at it this way—if it is cancer, you might end up getting a whole new set of breasts that look even better than the ones you have." She smiled and winked at me and added, "It can be all good if you look at it that way." In that moment, laying there feeling her hand intertwined with mine, I felt God's hand all over me. With tears in my eyes, I smiled back at her and felt my mindset shift and perspective change. I realized that if I *did* have cancer, that I would make this scary, tragic diagnosis work to my advantage in every way imaginable. I decided right then and there that I would squeeze every bit of goodness from this experience and that I would win no matter what the outcome. I wasn't going to let cancer TAKE from me, I was going to let it GIVE to me.

It was Friday morning March 3, 2017, I'm sitting at a conference table with my co-workers waiting on a parent meeting to begin. My phone vibrates and I see "Dr. Davis' name pop up. I quickly excuse myself and step into an empty office next door. The doctor tells me that my tumor is malignant. She says it has not moved to my lymph nodes as far as she could tell, but that would have to be verified by further tests. She tells me I will be scheduled to see the breast surgeon to inform me of next steps. I hang up, go back to my meeting. I am numb and in disbelief. I sit through a 45- minute meeting. My mind is racing, but I'm not scared. I don't feel sad. I really don't feel much. As soon as the meeting was over, I rushed to my office and close the door. I sat in my black swivel office chair and just stared at the wall. I felt relatively calm because I had mentally prepared for this moment. I called my husband then other close family members. I do not remember what they said. My diagnosis was stage 1 invasive ductal carcinoma or in other words a malignant tumor. This simply meant that the cancer was in the early stages but had spread to the surrounding breast tissue. Thank God, that I found this lump early and the cancer had not spread to any other areas of my body. It is so important ladies to get regular mammograms and do your own self breast exams every month. Also know your family history and pass this information on to your children. Being proactive against breast cancer is the best way to beat it. I put on the armor of God and prepared for the fight of my life. I said to myself "game on, let's go!" I felt this was one of many challenges that I had faced over the years and had always won in the past. Now, it was time to once again rise up and face this trial with all of the tools that God had equipped me with over the years. I prayed and believed that everything would be ok. At one point, I even told myself that even if I die, I still win. As crazy as it sounds, I knew I would win because of the testimony and legacy I would leave behind, through my fight. I believed that if God chose to let me die, I would go out like the champion that He created me to be and that I would undoubtedly bless someone in the process; not only by how I fought, but how I glorified Him to the very end. I was ready for whichever way this thing went. As I began to share my secret; my friends, family and colleagues were amazed by how I was handling my situation. Through pitiful glances, blank stares and bone-breaking hugs, they admired my strength, confidence and bravery. Little did they know that my battle had almost become an invigorating challenge for me in a strange kind of way. It was as if I had been given this unique test, for which it was an honor to be chosen. I was excited to exercise all of the wisdom and faith I had acquired over the years. Again, I had the full armor of God on and was ready for battle.

A few weeks after my diagnosis, I was given the option of either having a lumpectomy with radiation or a double mastectomy with no radiation. A lumpectomy would simply remove the tumor and surrounding tissue and the radiation would kill any of the cancer that may have spread to my surrounding breast tissue. The thought of radiation or chemo scared me more than having both my breast removed. I had heard so many negative things about those treatments that the thought of it made me cringe. My genetic tests were negative for the BRACA 1 and BRACA 2 gene, making a mastectomy optional, but not necessary. If a woman tests positive for the genetic mutation BRACA 1 or BRACA 2, the risk for developing breast cancer is very high. That's why many women, like celebrity Angelina Jolie, choose to have a double mastectomy prior to having a cancer diagnosis. Instead, my doctor gave me the choice on which way I wanted to go and didn't lean towards one option versus the other. Getting just the lumpectomy would leave me with one slightly smaller breast than the other and all of the uncomfortable side effects of the radiation. My other choice was to have a double mastectomy with no radiation and a reduced threat of ever having breast cancer again. The benefit of this option was that I could have two new smaller, perkier reconstructed breasts—the breasts of my dreams and no more mammograms. For me, the choice was simple and with my husband's blessing, I opted for the double mastectomy; after all, my sex appeal and womanhood were not defined by my breasts—so it was an easy choice.

Ladies, do not be afraid of a mastectomy if that is what you need to be healthy and cancer free. With the new technology and reconstruction techniques, your breast can look and feel better than the old ones. Yes, you can keep your nipples if the cancer has not spread to that area or you can get a reconstructed nipple with a 3D areola tattoo. A lot of women want to know if they will have any feeling or sensation in their breast—some do and some do not. It depends on the type of mastectomy and reconstruction that you have. These are questions that should be discussed with your health care provider prior to making any decisions regarding your treatment. Trust me, it's possible to look beautiful and sexy after a mastectomy, but that will depend on your specific procedure and doctors. Nothing is guaranteed. Mark's reassurance that he would support my decision and love me regardless of my choice, was all of the confirmation I needed that God had truly blessed me with the perfect soulmate and teammate!

Now that my diagnosis was proclaimed, and my treatment plan was finalized, it was time to tell my daughters. My oldest, Somer, was 20 at the time and in college out of state. When I made the call to her, I had to make sure that the words and my tone were upbeat and optimistic as not to alarm her. She was too far away from home to properly comfort her as only a mother could. After telling her about the discovery of the lump in my breast and how it was nothing to be worried about, I paused long enough for her to ask, "So you have cancer Mom?" I was caught red-handed so replied with a simple, "Yes." She remained silent for a few seconds more, but from the hundreds of miles and optic waves away, I could feel her energy. When I heard her sobbing through the phone, I instantly went into Mommy-mode, reassuring her that I would be ok and that I wasn't going to die. Sydney, on the other hand, was 15 at the time and a freshman in high school. She had always been "tough as nails" on the exterior, but "softer than butter," on the interior. Sydney didn't have quite the same reaction, but I kept close watch over her in the days to follow in case her behavior changed. As my surgery date got closer, she had the meltdown I was expecting. Her Dad ended up calling me to tell me that she broke down to him and admitted that she thought I was going to die. As much as I tried to reassure her that God was going to heal me, she just couldn't process the fact that her Mommy had cancer. The poem I share at the beginning of the book, "Weight on Your Shoulder," describes her feelings during her ordeal. She wrote it shortly after my surgery. It still leaves me in awe every time I read it.

Disclosing my diagnosis and treatment plan to the rest of my family gave me unimaginable peace. I didn't discuss "it" much after that because with each mention, it became harder and harder to vocalize. I couldn't say the word—CANCER. Instead, I would use subtle substitutes, like "the tumor," "the C," or "it"—anything but cancer. I didn't want to talk about it; instead, I just wanted it to be over so that I could get back to my life and my wedding planning. For a brief moment, the thought crossed my mind that my diagnosis was my punishment for divorcing my husband, and father of my children. The devil wanted me to believe that this was my payback for going against God's word, but I knew better. Instead, I knew that this "lesson" would once again be my blessing—I allowed the power of positive thinking to seep into my brain and it prevailed, once again.

Before I knew it, it was mid-March and I faced with the decision of either having the wedding and honeymoon we had planned for in May or postponing my surgery until after the wedding. Mark wouldn't hear of it and insisted that my health came first and that we needed to take care of "it" as soon as possible. I knew that my treatment plan would include a double mastectomy along with removal of some lymph nodes and if my lymph nodes were positive, I would then have to undergo radiation or chemo. If I had to have chemo/radiation, the breast reconstruction surgery would be next and the process from beginning to end could take months.

There were just so many unknowns that I decided to postpone the wedding. There was no possible way I could make plans based on when or if I would be healthy enough to get married; let alone travel. God's favor prevailed in that I was able to get a full refund for our flights to Hawaii as well as our deposit from the wedding venue. This allowed me to re-focus all of my efforts and energy on the battle that still lie ahead. Although my load was lightened in a sense, I still couldn't shake the feelings of guilt for not just the postponement of the wedding but for having cancer period. In the back of my mind, I couldn't help but to wonder how Mark really felt about the whole ordeal and if his feelings for me had changed in light of everything we had gone through thus far. I also questioned if he would look at me differently in the physical sense and if he would still be attracted to me without my real breasts. Millions of negative thoughts popped into my head and as much as I tried to control them and block them out, I couldn't help but to wonder how my situation would change things between us and if he still even wanted to marry me.

After all, this was not what he signed up for and he would be well within his right to leave if it was too much for him to handle. Without warning, my emotions took over and I became an emotional basket-case and subconsciously began to push him away. One minute I told him we shouldn't get married until the whole ordeal was over with and the next minute I told him we needed to go to the Justice of the Peace right away and get it over with. No matter what I said, he was fine with it and remained a rock the entire time, making it hard for me to ascertain how he really felt. The more I prayed, the more peace prevailed and allowed me to remain steadfast in my decision to get married as soon as I was feeling up to it. I refused to let the enemy steal my joy—the joy that God had promised me; had promised US.

I had my bi-lateral mastectomy on April 24, 2017. My entire family was there, with the exception of Somer who was away at college, and a lot of Mark's family as well. Even though I told Mark he did not have to stay with me, he was there all three nights sleeping on the uncomfortable hospital couch in my room, which reconfirmed for me the type of man God had blessed me with; a man who would soon be my husband. The surgery itself went well with no complications and the support I received during my recovery was unfathomable. My sister used most of her vacation time to stay with me during my recovery. Between Katina, Mark and other family members, they made sure I was fed, medicated and that I made it to all of my follow-up appointments. I couldn't have wished for a better support system. I had two procedures and two doctors during my first surgery. The breast surgeon performs the mastectomy then the plastic surgeon places temporary tissue expanders in the breast pocket immediately after the mastectomy. The expanders slowly stretched my skin in preparation for my new implants. Ladies, you can pick any size you want, always look for your silver lining.

While I was somewhat insecure about the removal of my breasts, I knew no one could tell through my clothes that I had undergone a bi-lateral mastectomy, so I decided that I could get married because I would still look good in my wedding dress. The hardest part was waiting for the lab results of my lymph node biopsy because if they were positive for cancer, I would have to undergo radiation or chemotherapy. As expected, my prayers were answered—the doctor gave me the good news that my lymph nodes were clear.

After it was evident that I was in the clear and on the road to recovery, my mom approached me about visiting Ma'Dea's old church, my original home church, to give my testimony about my ordeal. I was taken aback by her request and quickly declined it and told her that I didn't care to talk about my ordeal and didn't want to be portrayed as a victim or a poster child for cancer. And besides, I told her, I "didn't want folks all in my business." At first, my refusal seemed to really hurt my mom. She expressed her disappointment and confusion about why I didn't want to share the fact that God had spared me and given me such a mighty blessing. In my mind, however, I felt that God had given me a test that I had passed with flying colors and with that I just wanted to focus on getting my new breasts, getting married, going to Hawaii and then getting back to work. In retrospect, I couldn't see my arrogance and my pride in foolishly believing that I was responsible for my own fate and survival through my ordeal.

About six weeks after my mastectomy, I started to feel better and almost back to my normal self, which prompted my decision that it was time to get the show on the road and get married! I didn't want to delay marrying my King and my ordeal had made me realize that it wasn't about the fancy wedding or the honeymoon—instead it was about the marriage and the vows we would be making to one another to stay the course, in sickness and in health. I made peace with the fact that because of my limited mobility, I would have to forego my dream vacation. So, on June 8, 2017 we were married. I wore a beautiful mermaid white strapless wedding dress and a long veil. I felt beautiful and it was truly one of the happiest days of my life. My wedding planner decorated the venue with fresh pink and red rose petals and candles down the aisle. The day was perfect with the exception of my Dad not being there to walk me down the aisle. He was in the hospital and was not going to be released in time to make it. Other than that, I was very proud of the fact that I was able to put together such a beautiful wedding and reception in only a few weeks. I was happy, in love and recovering. In my heart of hearts, I believed that I had weathered the storm and was emerging from the wilderness...

Blessing Lesson #7

Whenever you are faced with a life challenge, one of the first things you should do is ask yourself "How can I use this to personally grow, or to be a blessing to someone else?" When I was first diagnosed with cancer, I thought it was just for me—to grow closer to God. In reality, it was not only for me, but to be a blessing to someone else. Most of the trials we go through is not just for yourself, it's for those around you as well. Sometimes God will divide and subtract from you in order to add and multiply to you. I had all of these big plans for my wedding and honeymoon, and I was a little upset at first that this was all happening to me at this time in my life. I learned who was really in control and it wasn't me despite my meticulous and detailed planning. You will get thorns in your side as you travel this road called "Life." When you get a thorn in your side, pull it out and use it as a weapon to win your battles. Make sure you make your trials your footstool. Your attitude and outlook on life's disappointments can either make you better or worse. You have a choice in how you react to any situation. Choose the reaction that will help you and benefit you. It's a paradigm shift that has to take place to receive your full blessing. Begin practicing this new way of thinking on small things then graduate to big things. I'm thankful and blessed that Mark was right by my side and loved me regardless of my illness. But let me tell you—if he had decided to bolt, I would have thanked God for showing me this man's true colors before I married him. Of course, I would have been devastated and hurt which is a normal human emotion, but I would have also understood the bigger picture. Always look past your circumstances so you can see the blessings ahead.

THOUGHT PROVOKER #7:

Have you ever had a life changing event that you thought you could never recover from? Have you ever had a trial so big that it kept you from thanking and loving God? What did you learn from your previous trials and how will you use those lessons in future trials?

_____

_____

_____

_____

_____

_____

_____

_____

_____

_____

_____

_____

_____

_____

_____

Chapter 8

FULL CIRCLE

For I know the thoughts that I think toward you, says the Lord,
thoughts of peace and not of evil, to give you a future and a hope.
~Jeremiah 29:11~

No sooner than I began to settle into the state of normalcy that I had dreamed of achieving for nearly half of my adult life; the sky opened up and all hell broke loose in my life again. Just weeks after my wedding, one of my closest friends since college, Wytaine, passed away un-expectantly.

As I mentioned in Chapter 3, Wytaine and I were the type of friends that were always there for each other, no matter what. Because we lived on opposite ends of town, we didn't see each other much, but when we did it was like we skipped a beat. The last conversation we had was through text messaging when I reached out to make sure she received my wedding invitation. She confirmed receipt and stated that she'd be attending; so, when she didn't show up, I figured something came up. I had full intentions on calling her to follow-up and of course wanted to give her a hard time about being a "no show," but I never did.... Imagine my shock when I got the call that she was in the hospital on life support—days later she was gone.

As the saying goes, when it rains, it pours. Within weeks of burying my best friend, I got the call from Mark that he had been laid off from his job; the very same job that had doubled his salary just twelve months prior. I couldn't believe it! Mark had literally given this company all of his time, efforts and energy for the last 12 months. He worked 12-hour days nearly six days a week. Thankfully, Mark seemed unbothered—his hustler mentality kicked in and he reassured himself and me that he would be back working in no time and within 2 days he was back at work.

With everything I had just endured, this temporary set-back paled in comparison; besides, I trusted God to take care of our needs. My faith was unwavering and finding a church home at Journey of Faith Baptist Church in Red Oak was what we needed to feed our faith and pull us through this latest ordeal. And it did, Mark was blessed with a new, better opportunity. Praise God! Nearly three months after my mastectomy, I had breast reconstruction surgery and I returned back to work in two weeks, even though I could have taken longer, I was anxious to get back to my job. All of my surgeries had been completed and thankfully, I did not need chemo or radiation, so it was time to dive back into work; besides, I loved my job and missed the interaction with my colleagues.

Five days after I returned to work from 2 major surgeries, our entire staff received notification of a district-wide Reduction in Force (RIF) due to budget constraints. At first, I wasn't concerned; instead I pulled from my "Faith Files" and based on everything I had been through, I knew I would be OK whichever way it went– besides, I knew that I had given my all for the last 4 years for this employer. I was that employee that always came to work and did my job to the best of my ability. All of my reviews were excellent. Boy, was I wrong.

Not too long after the announcement, the email came confirming that my role was included in the RIF. I was in shock and thought, *how could they do this to me with all I've been through?* What was even more shocking was that I was not offered the opportunity to transfer into another position and that two newer people with less experience in my department, were kept on. I had always exceeded expectations on my performance reviews and received rave reviews from my superiors and subordinates so I didn't know why this was happening to me.

Thoughts of discrimination, due to my condition, crept into my mind; especially given the fact that I was let go just five days after my return from medical leave. But once again, my unwavering faith kicked in, and I decided and trusted God to fight this battle too even though I had attorneys that wanted to take my case. Mark and I both believed that God would take care of us and anyone who purposefully did us wrong, so I moved on.

As I started my job search, I prayed that God would use this minor setback as an opportunity for me to explore other areas that I had put off exploring for fear of leaving my comfort zone. When a position for Behavioral Coach at a large school district popped up on the radar, I believed this was the job for me—not only did I meet all of the qualifications; but the job description matched what I was doing in my previous job. After weeks when I didn't hear back from them, discouragement set in once again.

While my doctor's appointments were dwindling down, with the exception of a routine checkup or two, I was referred to an oncologist who reviewed my genetic tests results and told me that the genetic tests I took back in March showed that I had the gene mutation called CDH1, which presented a 80% risk of stomach cancer. Needless to say, I was floored. *Not again Lord*, I thought. The doctor told me I would have to meet with a genetic counselor to review the details and get more information, one of which could be removal of the entire stomach if I did get cancer.

I left his office in tears and was distraught to the point that I couldn't even talk to God. I literally had no words. All of the optimism and faith that had carried me through to this point had diminished with one simple word—cancer. As much as Mark tried to keep me calm and comfort me, nothing worked. For the weeks leading up to my follow-up appointment with the genetic counselor, I couldn't help but to wonder if every little pain I felt in my stomach was cancer. I was absolutely miserable—it was all too much for me! In a six-month time span I had dealt with a breast cancer diagnosis, two major surgeries, loss of a friend, loss of two jobs, and the high possibility of getting stomach cancer. Then it happened.

It was a typical Sunday morning, September 17, 2017; but that particular morning something was different, something was off. I was tired. I was tired of pretending that I was ok. I was tired of fighting trial after trial. I was tired of being the strong wife, mother, daughter and sister. I was tired of being optimistic. I was tired of forcing a smile that wasn't there. Plain and simple—I was sick and tired. In an effort to get ready for church, I wandered lifelessly into the bathroom to get dressed. Mark was his usual, chipper, talkative self but even he could tell that something was wrong with me. It took everything in me to force responses to his questions and comments out of my mouth. My spirit was at an all-time low; so much so that I considered skipping church; but Mark insisted that we go.

An hour later, I walked aimlessly into church and forced a smile to onlookers as we took our seats. My body was there, but my mind was anything but. I couldn't even fake it anymore—my spirit wouldn't let me clap or pray or even force out an Amen during the sermon. When church was over, I didn't stop to fellowship but instead made my way to the car and plopped down in the seat, relieved that it was over. When we got home, my legs felt weak as I walked into our home. As soon as I made it to the bedroom, I laid across the bed in my full church garb. Now, Mark knew something was wrong because my clothes were usually the first things that came off whenever I got home from church or anywhere. When he asked me if I was ok, I fought back tears and told him I just wanted to rest.

After several more minutes of just lying there, I got up, changed into my loungewear and made my way to the kitchen. Every step I took, felt like I had a ton of bricks in each leg. I leaned over and grabbed a pot from the lower cabinet, gripping the counter hard as not to lose my balance. Upon opening up the top cabinets to reach for my measuring cup, I suddenly stopped, rested both hands on the granite countertop below me and dropped my head in despair. I didn't understand what was wrong with me. It was like no other feeling I had experienced. The weight was getting heavier and heavier. Tears begin to well up in my eyes.

At that moment, Sydney walked into the kitchen and asked, "Momma, what's wrong?"

Without hesitation, I turned my face and replied, "Nothing baby." I didn't want her to see me crying.

Once she had disappeared back into her room, I started to pace back and forth in the kitchen. I needed something, but didn't know what. I couldn't hold it in any longer—the last six months of my life had been a living hell; despite the show of optimism, faith and hope I tried to put on for those around me. In that moment, I felt myself being broken all the way to the point where I could no longer function and knew I had to release all of the pain, hurt and loss I had bottled up. I felt like I needed a good, loud, dry-heaving cry. I needed to cry not only for the loss of my breasts, but for the loss of my friend, the loss of my job and the loss of my hope as a result of being told I could possibly have stomach cancer!

I moved quickly into the garage and got into the driver's seat of my car. I slammed the door and let the darkness of the garage surround me as I prepared to have the cry of my life. Expecting the tears to flow, I gripped the steering wheel and pressed my forehead against it, determined not to let Mark or Sydney hear what was about to come out. I was ready to release all of the tears that my heartache had to offer but tears never came. In my confusion and frustration, I began to cry out to God!

"What do you want from me? I have tried to do everything you asked of me! I have been faithful to your word and believed in you for your blessings! What in the world do you want from me?"

I want you. God's voice came suddenly, in the form of a whisper that caressed my heart and soothed the anger that was boiling up inside of me. He had my full attention. **Yes, you have been faithful, but you won't tell anybody about all of the things I've done for you. You don't want to share the goodness of me; you choose to keep it all to**

yourself. Tell people what I can do and what I've done. That's all I've wanted. That's all I've ever wanted...

In an instant, the heaviness and hopelessness that was weighing me down, immediately left my body. I got out of the car and returned to the kitchen. I had emerged from the darkness of my garage into the light. God's words to me had cleared the path for me towards my purpose and everything now made sense. He wanted to use ME—what an honor! I knew what I had to do.

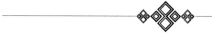

Blessing Lesson #8

We've all heard the saying that God will not put more on you than you can bare. Well, let me tell you when life situations feel too heavy to bare, that's when you're forced to turn it over to God. Sometimes that's the only way He can get your attention. When I look back over my life, I realize, like all of us, that I have made some mistakes and wrong turns. There are things that have happened to me because of my bad decisions, and there are things that I had no control over. If I could go back and change anything in my past, I wouldn't change a thing. Everything that has happened to me has made me who I am today. I'm stronger, wiser and ever more grateful. When you have Jesus in your life, you don't have to fear anything. It doesn't matter how bad it looks God is bigger than any of it. When you try to carry all the burdens on your shoulders, it will break you down and make you weak. Out of your weakness you will become stronger. You don't know how weak you are until you try to lift something heavy. That's why you have trials—to get stronger!

THOUGHT PROVOKER #8:

Has God ever told you to do something and you didn't do it? Have you ever had that nagging feeling deep inside you that you were supposed to be doing something other than what you are doing? What is He telling you to do?
Why haven't you been obedient?
What do you think will happen if you never step out on faith and do what's in your heart?

_____

_____

_____

_____

_____

_____

_____

_____

_____

_____

_____

EPILOGUE

It is not by chance that God spoke to me back in 2003, on September 18th and then again on September 17th, 2017; which is almost 15 years to the date. He told me then that I would be a "light in someone's dark world," but I had no idea what he meant at the time. He also promised that my life would be beautiful and that my "cup would overflow"—and He has been faithful on both counts! Nearly three weeks after my second cancer scare, Mark and I walked out of the hospital holding hands and smiling, after being told that my potential stomach cancer had been misdiagnosed. As if that wasn't blessing enough, a week after the breakdown in my garage, I started my new job as a Behavioral Coach; a role which I still hold to this very day.

The following Sunday, I returned to church; only this time I was on a mission. When Pastor Johnson announced that it was "testimony time," I knew I had to tell my story. Despite my uneasiness, stemming from my inherent fear of public speaking, God's words reverberated in my head and my heart—"tell the people about my grace and mercy," He said, and so I did. My voice was shaky and there were tears in my eyes as I poured into the congregation and shared with them everything I had experienced and how God had brought me through it all. Since this time, God has opened up doors which have allowed me to share my testimony numerous times. He has also convicted me to share His goodness with the masses, in the form of this book, which I hope has blessed you. "If you don't write this book, there may be someone out there that will not be saved, He said. "And if you only help one person from telling your story, my purpose for you will have been served—remember, it's not about you, but about others."

In closing, if there is one thing I would leave you with is that wherever you are in life is where you are supposed to be; meaning whether you are sick, unemployed, suffering a loss or being abused —no matter the trial you are experiencing, just know that you are exactly where you're supposed to be in that moment. After all, the trials we go through in life is what makes us stronger and allow us to glorify God at the same time. Thinking back to all of the trials I've endured in my life, from my molestation as a child, to being spared from a potential rape and possibly death, I now know that none of them were by accident. It wasn't until I learned to look at every bad situation as a stepping stool and not a punishment or an admonishment from God. When I started thanking Him for my problems and believing that they were going to work to my advantage is when I realized the power and strength that God placed inside of me—He has placed it inside of each one of us.

Just remember, God is faithful to His promises. He never promises us a life without pain and heartache, but He does promise you peace if you seek Him and his Kingdom. God had to break me all the way down to my knees for me to realize this. He had to humble me and let me know who He is. I thought I was doing everything right, but when God has a plan for you, he will move mountains and open doors that you never imagined could be opened. He will give you strength and courage you never knew you had. He will place the right people in your path and remove the wrong ones. I am so thankful to Him for using me as His vessel and for showing me how to turn my lessons learned into my blessings. Trust me, you don't have to be perfect—I am certainly not, but I do trust Him and allow Him to be God. It is only when you do this that He will give you the *Peace* of mind that is required to ignite your *Passion* to serve and glorify Him. This, and only this, will ultimately lead you to your *Purpose.* Thank you for allowing me to share it with you.

ACKNOWLEDGMENTS

First, I would like to thank my personal Lord and Savior Jesus Christ for choosing me to deliver His message. Everything I have and everything I am is because of Him. I would like to personally thank the following individuals who has supported and loved me throughout my life lessons.

To my husband **Mark Mingo**, thank you for being strong and supportive throughout my cancer battle. Your love and strength was everything to me. Thank you for supporting my dreams and goals in writing this book. You have always believed in me, even when I didn't, so thank you my love. Thank you, **Mya Mingo**, for being the sweetest, kindest step-daughter a person could ask for.

To my daughters **Somer and Sydney Lewis**, you girls were so strong and poised when you learned about my cancer diagnosis. Even though you may have been scared, you were able to pull it together and keep moving forward. I am proud of how strong and independent you are. I appreciate you all listening to all of my dreams over the years and being honest in your opinions. Thank you for the love and joy you have brought to my life.

To my parents, **James and Lura Hawkins**, thank you for providing me with so much love and security growing up. You provided an environment for me that allowed me to grow and flourish into the woman I am today. Your support and prayers during my cancer was a blessing to me, and I love you for that.

To my grandparents **Isaac and Mineola Burleson (Ma'dea)**, thank you for caring and loving me. The spiritual foundation you laid for me will carry on for generations. You taught me how to love people and love God. You taught me strong work ethic and how to fight through your storms. Because of you, I am here. I know that you are smiling down at me from Heaven. I am eternally grateful and will always love you!

To my sister, **Katina Baldwin**, you are a best friend and sister all rolled into one. I thank God that mama gave me a baby sister. You have always been there for me whenever I needed you. We have laughed and cried together all of our lives. Thank you for all the sacrifices you made to be here with me while I recovered from cancer treatment. Your prayers and support was truly a blessing for me. You are one-of-a-kind!

To my aunt, **Erma Murphy**, thank you for being a 2nd mom to me. You have been there since the beginning and have loved and supported me my entire life. You always made sure I had what I needed, all I had to do was ask. You sent me money and care packages all through college. I don't know how I would have made it without you.

To my niece, **Paige Hawkins**, I have loved you since the day you were born. You inspire me with your amazing work ethic and creativity. Watching you start several businesses as a teenager has inspired me to reach for the stars. You believe that you can do anything.....and you can. Thank you for being the best niece ever.

To my closest friends and family **Sabrina McCullough, Ebony Lawson-Brumfield, Pat Piper** and **Dana Mingo**. Thank you for being there for me whenever I needed you. I'm truly grateful to have friends and family that love me the way you do. You were right there by my side through my cancer and just knowing that you were there for me warmed my heart and healed my body.

To **Angie Ransome-Jones,** thank you for taking me under your wing and mentoring me through this entire process. You have guided me from beginning to end and I am ever so grateful. Thank you for always giving me honest feedback and never being afraid to tell me the truth. The books you have written has inspired me to write, and I could not have done this without you.

To **Superintendent and Pastor Robert Jackson and First Lady Angela Jackson** of Perry Memorial Church of God and Christ, thank you for giving me the very first opportunity to speak and share my story. You believed in me and gave me the confidence to stand before others and tell "my truth." I am forever grateful for you and **Reverend Lennard Ball**, as well as all of the members of Perry Memorial, who interceded upon my behalf during my cancer battle.

To **Pastor Willie R. Johnson and First Lady Marion Johnson** of Journey of Faith Baptist Church, thank you for welcoming Mark and I into your church family. Thank you for the love, support and prayers that you and your church family gave us from day 1. We are forever grateful.

ABOUT THE AUTHOR

Karla Mingo grew up in Bryan, TX and graduated from Bryan High School in 1987. She earned a Bachelor of Science degree in Criminal Justice from The University of North Texas and is currently pursuing her Master's degree in School Counseling from Walden University. Prior to her transition into the field of Education, Karla worked as an adult probation officer for ten years. With ten years of Education under her belt, Karla is currently employed as a Behavioral Coach at an elementary school in the Dallas/Ft. Worth area.

Karla is an active member of Journey of Faith Baptist Church in Red Oak, TX and a member of Circle of Hope Breast Cancer Support Group at Oak Cliff Bible Fellowship (OCBF) in Dallas, TX. In addition, she serves as Vice President of the non-profit/501C-3 organization My Sister's Keeper Coalition, an organization that mentors young women. Lastly, Karla is the Founder and President of Pink Heavenly Angels, a non-profit organization she founded in 2018, to assist women battling breast cancer. Karla, who is herself a breast cancer survivor, currently resides in the Dallas area. She is married to her husband Mark and has two daughters, Somer and Sydney.